Joy *of* Balance

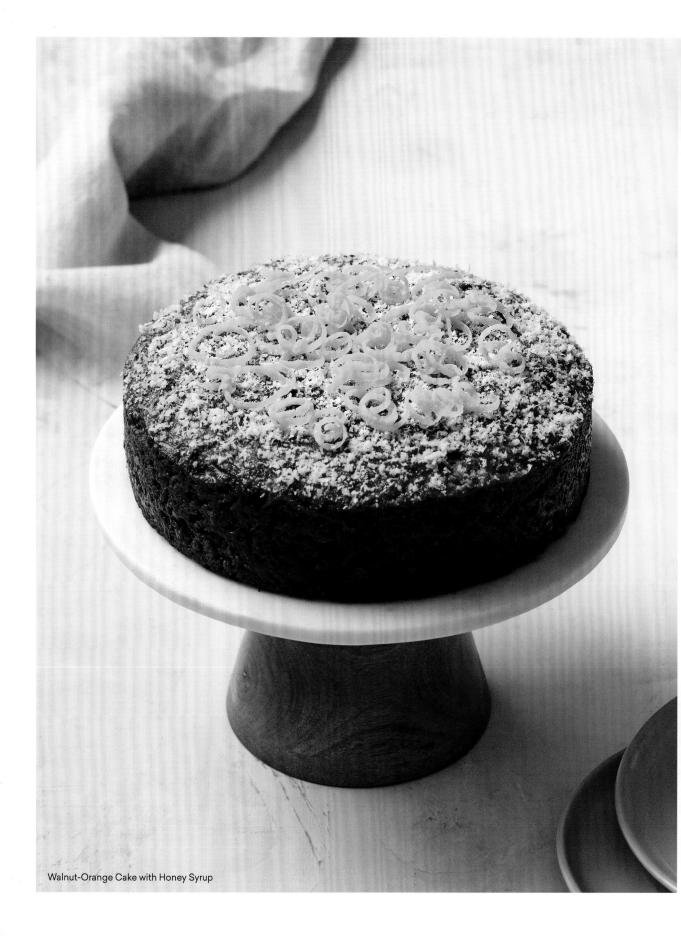

Walnut-Orange Cake with Honey Syrup

Joy of Balance

An Ayurvedic Guide to
Cooking with Healing Ingredients

—

80 PLANT-BASED RECIPES

Divya Alter

Photography by Rachel Vanni

RIZZOLI
NEW YORK

New York Paris London Milan

contents

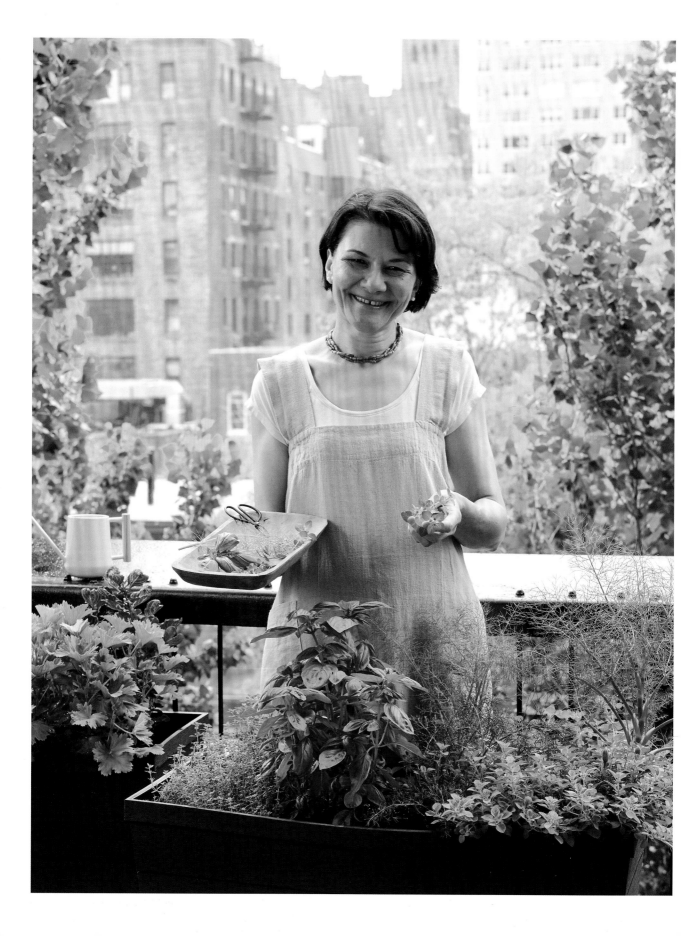

healing calls for a change

Healing calls for a change—a change in perspective, in habits, and in the way we interact with others. You can't force healing on yourself or someone else. Like creativity, healing has its own timing. And when the time is right, you will have the strength and determination to break up the known and unknown patterns that no longer serve your human evolution.

To me, healing the mind and body is a mysterious and courageous process, a lifelong journey with unexpected twists and turns. It often feels like I am being guided by a sublime plan that is beyond my comprehension. Before the body shifts, first the mind must change. I've undergone the deepest healing transformations during the most difficult, pleasure-lacking periods in my life. During such times of crippling fear and desperation, healing emerged when I was able to let go of attachment and worry while simultaneously forgiving and accepting who I am; I felt reborn.

"What is nature communicating to me? What am I supposed to learn from this situation? Can I find love right now?" I asked myself these questions many times during the year of 2020, when we all shared the unprecedented world turmoil caused by COVID-19. It was a time of painful uncertainty and global recalibration. As we remained confined in our homes for weeks and months, many of us reevaluated our lives, reset our priorities, and gained clarity on what to do next. Many of my friends who survived the virus felt as if they were given a second life. "I can breathe again. It's time for me to start over in a more wholesome way," a friend of mine shared as she celebrated her recovery from a six-week fight with the coronavirus. Although I was not infected with the virus, I, too, went through some significant healing shifts. This is when I envisioned the concept of *Joy of Balance* and started writing about it.

This book is the ingredient-driven sequel to my first cookbook, *What to Eat for How You Feel: The New Ayurvedic Kitchen* (Rizzoli, 2017), which, as of the time of writing, is in its ninth edition and has a German translation. My first book connected me with readers from all over the world and laid the ground for exciting opportunities. Since the publishing of that book, I've reflected on some lessons I've learned through the changes in my life.

my contentment:
through serving nourishing food

My mentor and dear friend Dr. Pratima Raichur (the founder of Pratima Skincare and Spa) advised me to use my cooking skills to nourish people, teach them to nourish themselves, and bring their hearts close to each other. These wise words have been a guiding principle in my career. I am a chef who cares about your gut and emotional health. Providing healing and nourishing food is where I find art in my life; it is how I try to serve and benefit others. It thrills me to know that the recipes I create or the dishes I prepare can contribute to a person's healing process by increasing their vitality and well-being.

divya's kitchen:
a business of service

In 2016, my husband, Prentiss, and I launched Divya's Kitchen, the first Ayurvedic restaurant in New York City. It quickly landed on OpenTable's 50 Best Restaurants for Vegetarians in America, was named the Best Healthy Restaurant in Manhattan and the Tri-State Area, and joined the list of 10 Best Overall Restaurants in New York City, an especially noteworthy ranking for plant-based cuisine.

The success of Divya's Kitchen did not come easy. Behind the glory, there was the "grind"—the exhaustion, occasional desperation, and long hours of hard work. If you've ever been an entrepreneur, you'll relate when I say that owning a business stretches your barriers, tests your faith, and pushes your buttons to their limits. But I would rather do what I love and grow through the challenges than force myself into a job that doesn't align with my life's purpose. For me, the most nurturing aspect of being a restaurateur is meeting our guests, watching them restore their energy, and connecting with our local community through events and programs such as small business owners' support groups and feeding the homeless. From the start, I realized that even though Divya's Kitchen carries my name and it represents who I am, the business is not just about me. It is about serving as a team to benefit others. I continue to learn how the inner disposition of service—in this case, through the mundane task of restaurant ownership—can become a catalyst for spiritual awakening.

pantry products:
a taste of divya's at your home

We had to close Divya's Kitchen during the first two months of the 2020 pandemic lockdown in New York City. Our regular customers, now forced to cook at home while adjusting to their new work and childcare arrangements, kept reaching out to us: "How can we quickly recreate Divya's food at home?" In response, Prentiss and I created a line of Ayurvedic pantry products aimed at providing an easy way to feel nourished and balanced every day. From several types of one-pot kitchari meals to soups and sauces, Divya's pantry products are a welcoming answer for our devoted customers: these products call only for water and twenty minutes of low-maintenance cooking (see Sources, page 248). The response nationwide was most encouraging. I am continuing to create more options for comforting on-the-go meals for any time of the day, in any season. I learned that when I desire to help people, new opportunities for service will arise, and I should not hesitate to take them.

ayurvedic culinary education: a passion to share

Helping others learn how to prepare wholesome meals at home is my favorite occupation. Teaching not only deepens my own understanding and practice of the ancient wisdom; it also brings me true joy as I interact with my students and observe their excitement from discovering wellness in their kitchen.

I firmly believe that health-supportive culinary education that teaches people how to prepare wholesome meals will reduce their and their loved ones' risk of numerous diet-related diseases such as diabetes, obesity, high cholesterol, gut inflammation, and heart failure. Studies show that people who cook at home will eat out less, and thus consume fewer bad fats, sugars, and ultra-processed foods. As my friend and one of the founders of Culinary Medicine, Chef Robert Graham, MD, would say, "Cooking for yourself is healthier and cheaper than not." There is no doubt that cooking at home equals better health; therefore, I dedicate a significant portion of my time to teaching, writing, and speaking publicly about how to make home cooking easy and fun.

During the past few years, we expanded the virtual and in-person programs of our nonprofit school, Bhagavat Life, to provide introductory and seasonal cooking classes, weekend immersive workshops, and a comprehensive two-level Ayurvedic Nutrition and Culinary Training (ANACT). We also continue to produce pre-recorded courses on healthful cooking and self-care, which can be accessed by anyone anywhere in the world (see Sources, page 248). Teaching is my humble offering of gratitude to my many teachers who have shaped and continue to shape my character and guide my path.

my continued ayurveda education: a lifelong endeavor

My Ayurveda teacher of the Shaka Vansiya (SV) lineage, Vaidya R. K. Mishra, suddenly passed away on the day my book *What to Eat for How You Feel* was released. I felt devastated. I knew that Vaidya continued to live through his teachings, and my connection with him was not lost, yet it took me about three years of grieving and acceptance before I could resume my Ayurveda education. Taking master classes at the DINacharya Institute led by Bhaswati Bhattacharya, MD, immensely expanded my knowledge of food and healing. In this book, I present a summary of what I've learned from my advanced studies with Dr. Bhattacharya and other teachers at the DINacharya Institute.

I also continue to learn a great deal from my collaborations with some of my heroes and leading experts in Ayurveda and wellness: Dr. Marianne Teitelbaum, Dr. Pratima Raichur, Krishna Kshetra Swami, Jai Dev Singh, Dr. John Douillard, Dr. Robert Graham, Ky Scott, Chef Richard LaMarita of the Institute for Culinary Education, and more. I am ever indebted to them for helping me deepen my knowledge and practice of Ayurveda and life in general. I learned that by cultivating my innate intuition, I can access the subtleties of human existence. I can live with better awareness of myself and my surroundings, notice the intricacies of nature, and feel more connected with it.

a modern woman with a time-tested message

In *What to Eat for How You Feel*, I summarize the essential principles of Ayurvedic cooking and share over one hundred seasonal recipes. Organizing *Joy of Balance* by ingredient is my way of empowering you to develop a deeper, exciting connection with whole, plant-based foods. While *What to Eat for How You Feel* sets the groundwork for living a holistic lifestyle, *Joy of Balance* invites you to apply an Ayurvedic lens as you focus on the specific produce, grains, nuts, seeds, lentils, and dairy that make up your meals. This approach will help you develop a more intimate relationship with the ingredients and satisfy you physically, mentally, and emotionally. You will be motivated to add my Millet Pilaf with Grated Carrots (page 60) to your spring meals when you learn how millet can bring you into balance—it resolves water retention in the body and scrapes impurities in the gut. It is tempting to want to experience the exceptional liver-cleansing and blood-sugar-lowering properties of bitter melon, but it is just as important to know when and why not to eat it. Reading about the varieties of leafy greens and how to prepare them for best nutrient absorption might answer your question about why raw kale makes you bloated at times.

The vegetarian- and vegan-friendly recipes and ingredient descriptions in this book are based on the principles of Ayurveda, the traditional health-care system of India. We cannot turn a blind eye to a holistic modality that has successfully treated people for thousands of years, a time long before modern medicine emerged. By taking the best wisdom of the past and bringing it forward, I show that food does not have to be reinvented. In fact, many of today's trendy foods have nourished humanity for centuries. But how do you prepare einkorn or spelt, red or basmati rice, cabbage or cauliflower, kulthi or red lentils, coconut or cashews, or milk or cheese so that you can digest them best and benefit fully from their nutrients? How can you enhance physiological functions in your body with the foods you consume? Is it possible to make healthy cooking from scratch less time-demanding? You will find the answers to these and more questions in the upcoming pages.

Joy of Balance is for those who seek nourishment and balance of the mind and body—the real purpose of food. A lot of people define themselves by what they don't eat. "I'm gluten free" or "I don't eat dairy" or "I don't cook meat." In our efforts to feel better, we try different diets and often end up unknowingly eating the wrong foods. The first step to discovering the best eating pattern for *you* is to identify your body-mind constitution, your digestive capacity, and the foods that *you* enjoy eating. If you pay attention, your body tells you when it can no longer handle the heavy proteins, fried foods, or sugary drinks. By expanding your knowledge of food from merely flavoring and cooking techniques to applications for health, you will feel more attuned and empowered. Balanced eating is not a fad diet but involves self-awareness, and that is why balance is a personal, evolving, and holistic concept. I hope that my recipes, ingredient by ingredient, will delight, sustain, and heal you, and in so doing, will give you a newfound freedom in the kitchen.

I felt compelled to use a few Sanskrit terms that denote key Ayurvedic concepts because often a one-word translation is impossible or incomplete. A Sanskrit word can have a spectrum of meanings in different contexts. To reduce a word to only one meaning in one context can lead to a limited perception or misunderstanding of Ayurveda. If you lose track of a Sanskrit term, refer to the Glossary on page 246.

join me at my table, join me in my dream

Meaningful conversations and radical change start at the table. *Joy of Balance* is your invitation to my table. Here you can turn toward the things that bring you healing and happiness. Prioritize balance over perfection. Express kindness through the food you prepare. Reach out to someone you love, invite them to your table, and offer them nourishing food. Soak up the mutual joy from the interaction.

I also invite you to dream with me: imagine that we treat our food and those who bring it to our table with the utmost respect and gratitude. Imagine the positive impact that wholesome, lovingly prepared meals can have on our bodies, our minds, and our community. Imagine that most people honor their own health as a precious gift to be kept and cherished. Healthy habits are contagious. By embracing your own healing process, you subconsciously activate the spread of these healing vibrations for global betterment.

If you feel ready to welcome healing change in your life, take a deep breath, smile, and meet me in the next chapter.

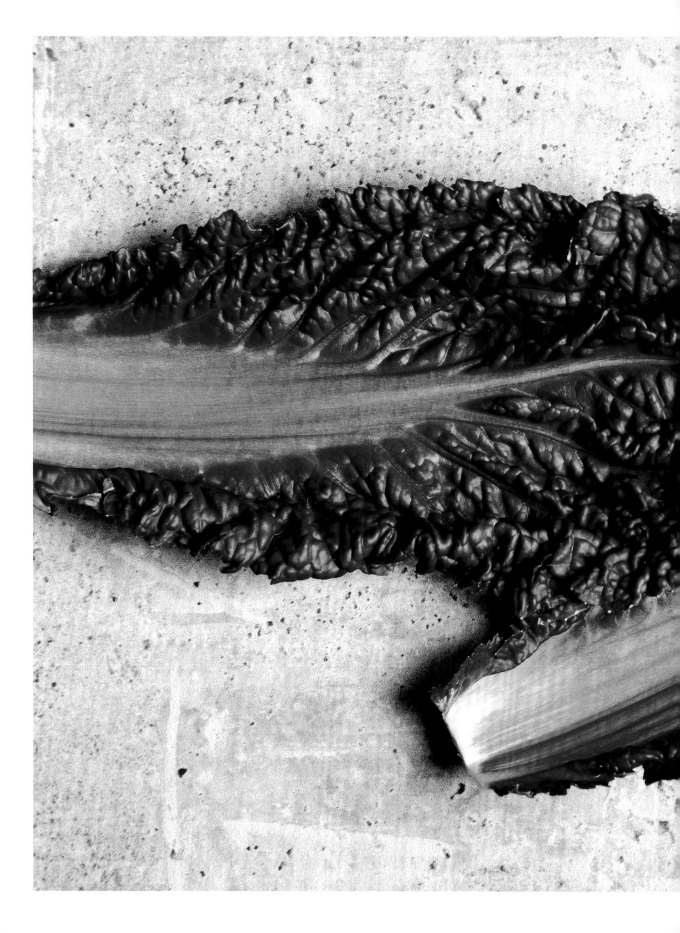

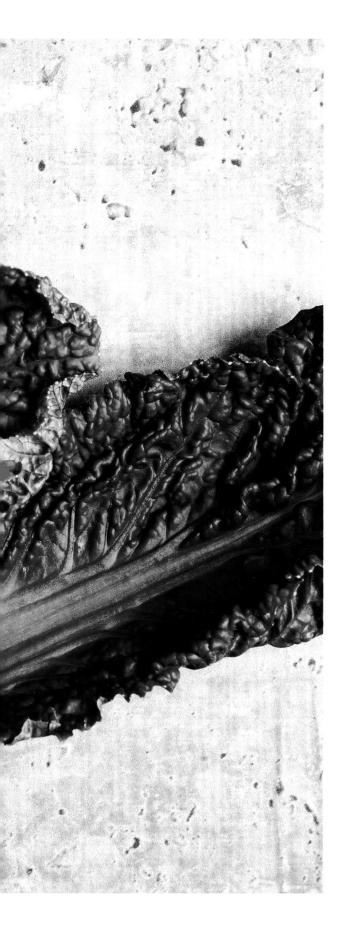

food
wisdom
from
ayurveda

For many years, I embraced the common perception that health is the absence of symptoms of disease. If my medical tests came out normal, I was considered healthy. But then I wondered: What about the times when I am not feeling well and yet all tests are normal? Am I still healthy, or is my sensation of dis-ease all in my head?

In my attempts to lead a healthier life, I gradually realized that maintaining good mental and emotional health is as important as physical health. It is no secret that suppressing the expression of what we're feeling leads to disease. It takes courage and self-love to open up to the world around us. Now more than ever, our cultural evolution underscores our human need for healthy expressions in a nonjudgmental community. What is the core concept that unifies us as humans and sets the ground for more acceptance and less judgment, creating a healthier environment for us to thrive? The ancient Vedic wisdom answers that.

As a health system, Ayurveda presents comprehensive knowledge of both preventative care and treatment of disease. Ideally, we want to apply Ayurveda as a way of life, not as medicine. However, if our lifestyle gradually breaks down our health, we have to seek help from a qualified Ayurvedic doctor and apply the medicinal aspects of this ancient practice.

Health trends and food fads come and go. However, Ayurveda has been around for centuries and is here to stay. Why? Because

Ayurveda presents the *principles* of life—the universal truths of preventative health care that can be applied by any person anywhere, at all times. These simple yet profound principles articulate nature's intelligence, and by following them intuitively, we can tune in to our own intelligence to choose what is good for our life right now. What's good is what will perpetuate health and happiness, and what's bad is what will decrease health and happiness. Furthermore, our needs change constantly, and everyone's needs are different. This subjective approach is extremely effective, but it can also be confusing if we don't have proper guidance.

Ayurveda gives us a systematic understanding of our interactions with nature. We humans are, too, living creatures of nature. We are as much a part of the ecosystem as the plants, animals, and insects we encounter around us. The difference is that those creatures are driven by nature's laws instinctively, without having free will to act and make choices. We have the conscious capability to choose our food, our lifestyle, and the environment we live in.

Here is one of Ayurveda's definitions of health mentioned in the two-thousand-year-old text called *Sushruta Samhita* (15.38):

A person is in good
health when he or she has

- balanced bio-elemental energies (a.k.a. doshas: Vata, Pitta, Kapha),

- strong digestion and metabolism,

- properly nourished and toxin-free body tissues (lymph, blood, muscle, fat, bones, bone marrow, reproductive fluids),

- timely formation and elimination of wastes (through urine, feces, and sweat),

- good coordination between the mind and senses, the mind and intellect, and the intellect and the soul, and

- happiness and contentment.

As you can see, Ayurveda's bar for health is pretty high! An expert Ayurvedic physician will evaluate your condition in all the above areas and search for the causes of dis-ease, not just address your symptoms. Keep in mind that we are designed to have a strong vitality and a calm mind, but we can't take them for granted. It's up to us to maintain the proper conditions for them to happen by taking care of our health daily. As an ancient saying goes, "A healthy person should be as vigilant to maintain good health as a sick person is as vigilant in curing their disease." On which side of the scale are you right now: maintenance or curing? Or are you neglecting both?

One of the ultimate goals of the Ayurvedic journey is to develop a subtle, spiritual receptivity to divine energy. This energy imbues our lives with deep meaning, and from this, we are capable of feeling a kind of bliss that is independent of our aging body. A genuine spiritual practice helps us connect with our eternal identity beyond the material realm. I find that daily yoga and spirituality allow me to access this subtle openness and lead a more soul-centered life. Such a life prepares us for the final lesson: to welcome death without fear, as a natural transformation and transition of the soul.

To live a purposeful, healthy, and happy life and to die without fear sounds like a dream, doesn't it? If you set it as a goal, with proper guidance, you can achieve it and it won't be only for your own sake. The closer you come to that goal, the more you will be able to increase happiness in the lives of others.

Ayurveda is here to help us heal. Healing unfolds gradually, and it involves our active participation. In my own healing journey, following Ayurveda's "rules" initially generated a lot of stress, which was definitely not healthy or Ayurvedic. I eventually learned an important lesson: Ayurveda's guidelines of what is good or bad for me are not meant to increase my rigidity and trap me mentally and emotionally while I try to do the right thing. Ayurveda is here to help us assess where we are and to flow with life. Its principles are a framework to guide us in developing our intuition and body wisdom about what is good or bad for our health.

Even though Ayurveda gives us a lot of information about body types and the dos and don'ts for each one of them, it is the opposite of a dogmatic or judgmental system. The fundamental Ayurvedic understanding is that we are all unique, and whether a food or herb is good for you or not depends on the conditions of your body and mind at the present time. Ayurveda truly embraces diversity, and thus applies a diverse, customized approach to healing each individual. Next, we will explore the source of this diversity, what makes up your unique constitution, and how to express it to promote healing.

prana: the cosmic energy, the elements, and the doshas

PRANA AND ITS COSMIC COMPONENTS

The topic of the origins of creation is a big and esoteric one. More recent philosophers and scientists continue to update their theories about where everything came from. The original *Vedas*, the Puranas, and the later Ayurvedic classical texts are among the oldest to outline detailed descriptions of how the material world manifested. For simplicity, most modern Ayurvedic explanations start with the five states of matter (often translated as the five elements) that make up planet Earth: ether, air, fire, water, and earth. But what is the source of these elements? The Shaka Vansiya Ayurveda lineage that I am a student of considers *prana* to be that source, a universal life force that consists of three components. And ultimately, *prana* originates from divine consciousness. The Ayurvedic philosophers came to this conclusion from their observations of *prana* and nature's interactions with the consciousness that occurs in creation.

The three main components of cosmic *prana* are the lunar energy (Soma), the solar energy (Agni), and the cosmic space energy (Marut). The Soma energy has specific effects on earth: it is cooling (have you noticed that temperatures drop around the time of the full moon?), stabilizing, and nurturing; it promotes growth and generates the taste in fruits and vegetables. The Agni energy is heating and brightening; it fuels all transformational processes on our planet. The Marut energy is the space and air that provide the container for the lunar and solar energies to circulate and interact. Marut is the subtle force that carries the grand intelligence behind creation's operations—it determines the paths of movement and the proportions of energetic transformations that constantly occur around us. The three energies coexist in a way that is analogous to a temperature control system in your house: it delivers cold or hot air (Soma and Agni, respectively), and the programmed thermostat (Marut) determines when to activate which temperature and for how long.

THE FIVE STATES OF MATTER AND THE THREE DOSHAS

The vibrational forms of Soma, Agni, and Marut manifest on a physical level as the five elemental energies or states of matter (commonly known as the five elements):

Prana has several interpretations. It can mean the cosmic subtle energy, which is the elementary biophoton particles of the sun and moon and their effects on everything on earth. In the words of Vaidya Atreya Smith, this type of *prana* is the energy that carries the potential of matter. *Prana* can also mean the life-giving energy that circulates in every living being and is the "thread" that keeps the body and soul together. Ayurveda defines life as the flow of *prana* in the body.

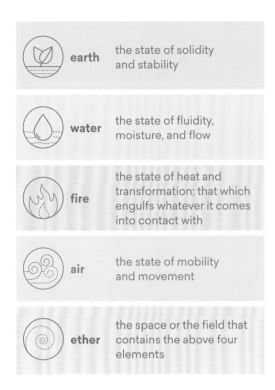

	earth	the state of solidity and stability
	water	the state of fluidity, moisture, and flow
	fire	the state of heat and transformation; that which engulfs whatever it comes into contact with
	air	the state of mobility and movement
	ether	the space or the field that contains the above four elements

Everything on earth is made of these elemental building blocks, and our relationship with them determines the level of harmony we have with nature. The five states of matter express themselves in the human body as the three doshas: Vata, Pitta, and Kapha (see diagram on page 18).

The term *dosha* has several meanings, and in the context of Ayurveda, it is often translated as "fault" or "weakness." The truth is, as with many Sanskrit words, it is hard to give a one-word English translation to this term. Dr. Bhaswati Bhattacharya helped me to understand its meaning in this way: Ayurveda views the body through functions (i.e., doshas); modern medicine relates to the body through form and structure. The doshas are *prana*'s energies that come into contact with the body (matter). They are the functions at play in human physiology—they work nonstop. Because matter constantly fluctuates, each dosha fluctuates and thus

becomes "that which creates imperfection." Anytime we do something in excess, our body systems and organs, "managed" by aggravated doshas, are subjected to pathology or disease.

To tie it all together, Soma, Agni, and Marut are the universal *prana* (macrocosm). These energies manifest into physical substance found in every aspect of the planet, creating the five states of matter, and these five states of matter combine to perform functions in the body (microcosm) by means of the Vata, Pitta, and Kapha doshas.

Vata dosha is the harmonious union of ether and air, and it takes on the qualities of these two elements in the body: dry, light, cold, rough, subtle, and mobile. Vata is the circulatory energy that governs the body-mind functions of movement, the nervous system, speech, breathing, elimination, sense of touch, creativity, and our innate healing intelligence; it also coordinates the movements of Pitta and Kapha.

Pitta dosha is the body's expression of the fire element protected by a smaller amount of fluidity (water element) and takes on their qualities: slightly oily (think of gasoline), penetrating, hot, light, slightly foul smelling, and spreading easily. Pitta is the "cooking energy" that governs transformation (all chemical and metabolic functions), digestion, body warmth, visual and mental perception, appetite, and thirst; it powers the intellect, luster, complexion, and courage.

Kapha dosha is the combination of the elements water and earth. When you mix them together, they turn into mud, and the Kapha qualities are very similar to those of mud: oily, cool, heavy, slow moving, moist, and stable. Kapha is the cohesive "glue energy" that provides structure, support, and static stability and makes up the bulk of bodily tissues. It maintains the functions of growth and provides nourishment and lubrication to the organs, tissues, joints, and

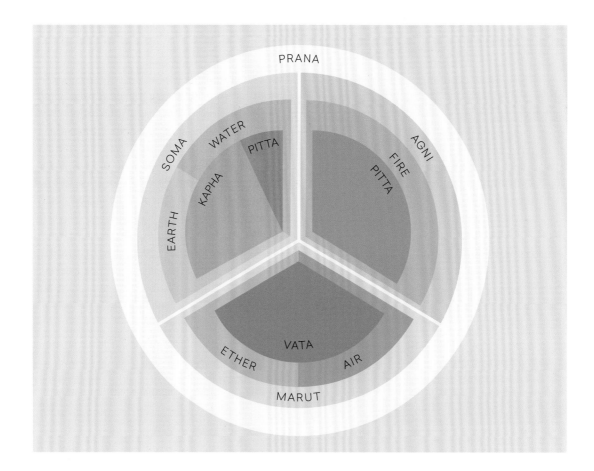

mucus membranes; it gives physical endurance and strength to the heart, lungs, brain, and other organs.

Vata activates when there is a need for something to move.

Pitta activates when there is a need for something to transform.

Kapha activates when there is a need for something to grow, lubricate, or be "cushioned" with protection.

All three doshas are present in everyone, but they express themselves in a unique way in each one of us. The distinctive combination of the doshas at our time of birth defines our constitution or natural disposition (*prakriti*). Most people have a predominance of one or two doshas, and some people have an equal amount of the three (tridoshic). The dominant dosha will be reflected in your self-expression: in the way you look, think, and operate in life. And that dominant dosha is usually the first one to go out of its optimal state when you're under stress.

The body is the landscape where the doshas interact to create either vitality or disease. You experience vitality when you are closest to your unique constitution and disease when you are furthest from it, a sign that your doshas are functioning abnormally. Too much Vata will create unnatural dryness, coldness, circulation and elimination issues, depletion, anxiety, fear, dissatisfaction, or insecurity. The overflow of Pitta will lead to excess heat, burning sensations, inflammation, impatience, impulsiveness, or anger. Excess Kapha will increase the feelings of heaviness, sluggishness, accumulation, inertia, lack of confidence, or sadness.

The doshas are bioenergies—we can't measure them with modern scientific tools. However, we can perceive them, just like we can perceive the mind's movements. And like all energy, the three doshas constantly fluctuate and "dance"—they are never static. Vata goes high when we're exercising, Pitta goes high when we're hungry, Kapha goes high when we're sleeping. However, in a healthy person, the heightened doshas become alleviated very quickly. In a dis-eased person, they accumulate, aggravate, and then displace themselves—this is when we begin to feel unwell.

It Is important to understand what your constitution, or metabolic type, is because it is your original blueprint for perfect health, and it guides you to proactively and continually maintain a healthy lifestyle. It is even more important to know how stress causes your current dosha dysfunction, the cause of your illness, or your feeling of being unwell. That dysfunction is what you need to correct to bring yourself back to your perfect health. Like it or not, for as long as you have a body and mind, you've got to deal with your doshas!

I love the concept of the doshas because it explains why we're all different and why we all have different needs. Knowing my constitution helps me align with my unique nature, better understand myself and my tendencies, and find my reference point for perfect health. This Ayurvedic concept also enables me to do the same with others, thus allowing me to feel more compassion. It reduces my judgmental habit of comparing myself to others and thinking that others should be like me. Now it is easier for me to discern when someone's self-expression stems from harmony, as a call *of* love, or from imbalance, as a cry *for* love, and from there, I look for a kind way to connect with that person.

If you'd like to find out your metabolic type and your imbalance, I encourage you

to refer to my first cookbook, *What to Eat for How You Feel*, where I elaborate on how the three doshas express themselves in their balanced or imbalanced states. In addition, there are many books on Ayurveda that dive deeply into these functional principles. And if you'd like to take it a step further but do not have a connection with an Ayurvedic doctor or practitioner, see Sources (page 248), where I list a couple of online "dosha quizzes" that I like. The fastest way to manage your doshas is with the right food. In the recipe section of this book, I will explain the effect that each featured ingredient or recipe has on the doshas.

You can use the concept of the doshas to learn so much about yourself: how your organism operates; identify its strengths and weaknesses; build true vitality for your own unique body; and provide real contentment for your own unique mind. Thus, you will lay a healthy terrain for accelerating your spiritual growth, which is the ultimate purpose of Ayurveda.

The components of *prana*, the five states of matter, and the doshas represent material energy. We—the soul—are of superior, spiritual energy, which can be perceived through our consciousness. For a long time, some of us have been existing in a somewhat unconscious, autopilot-like state, going through the motions of life while morphing ourselves into a personality that feels safe and secure. The Vedic practices help us increase self-awareness and become more conscious of who we are and what our unique purpose is. So don't just get stuck on the doshas; allow your Ayurvedic lifestyle to refine your mind and body so that you can tune in to the subtler and more powerful dimensions of human existence. This is when life gets interesting!

Now, let us discuss the connection between *prana* and food and how to select the foods that enhance your pranic flow, and thus your vitality, at any given time.

what is ayurvedic food?

For most of my life, I tried to eat healthful vegetarian food, or at least food that I thought to be healthful. Yet I could not understand why the cheese and smoothies I enjoyed in my twenties felt too heavy and unsettling in my thirties and forties. Isn't it that healthy food should always be healthy for me? How do I make the right health and wellness choices as I grow through the changes in life? Ayurveda answered all these questions in a way that made the most sense to me.

Many people ask me, "What is Ayurvedic food?" and in response I ask them, "What food is most balancing for *you, right now*?" Is celery juice Ayurvedic for you today, considering that it is astringent in taste, cooling, and it calls for higher digestive strength? If your Vata dosha happens to be out of balance and you're experiencing cold hands and feet, bloating, or a sense of being ungrounded, then no, celery juice is not Ayurvedic for you today. However, if your Pitta is high and you're agitated with acidic digestion, a burning sensation, or if you need a shot of alkalinizing fluid, then by all means, have a small glass of celery juice! I say a small glass because portion size also matters, but more on that later.

"Ayurvedic food" is the food that is most suitable for maintaining optimal health in the context of your appetite, dosha imbalance, physical activity, geographic location, the time of day or year, the time in your life, or the health condition you're experiencing. Ayurvedic food is not a set diet, but an evolving, personalized way of eating aimed at maintaining balance or overcoming a disease.

the golden rule of balance

There is an implicit law of nature that applies to us all: like increases like and opposites balance. When it's cold and windy outside, we seek warm shelter to alleviate the coldness and airiness in our body. In the scorching sun, we feel hot and look for a cool place to replenish ourselves. We all effortlessly follow this law in our relationship with the environment, but less so in our relationship with food. It takes a bit more effort to learn how to determine the food that balances you because you need to acquire basic knowledge of how different foods interact with the human organism. And so, most of us eat the way we learned at home, which often isn't the healthiest way.

When I was younger and less "conscious," I didn't really care much about my food selection. I just picked food available to me because I was hungry. In time, I started experiencing more and more digestive issues that one day woke me up with a definitive yet somewhat scary message: "Something's wrong."

We've all had that feeling in relation to some aspect of our health. That is natural, but where do you go from there? Ayurveda reveals that we have a threshold of vitality within our senses. Once we cross it, we enter the realm of misusing or overusing our senses, and our body starts to send us signals: "I can't endure that anymore!" Getting to that point is the perfect time to reevaluate and reset the way we eat and live.

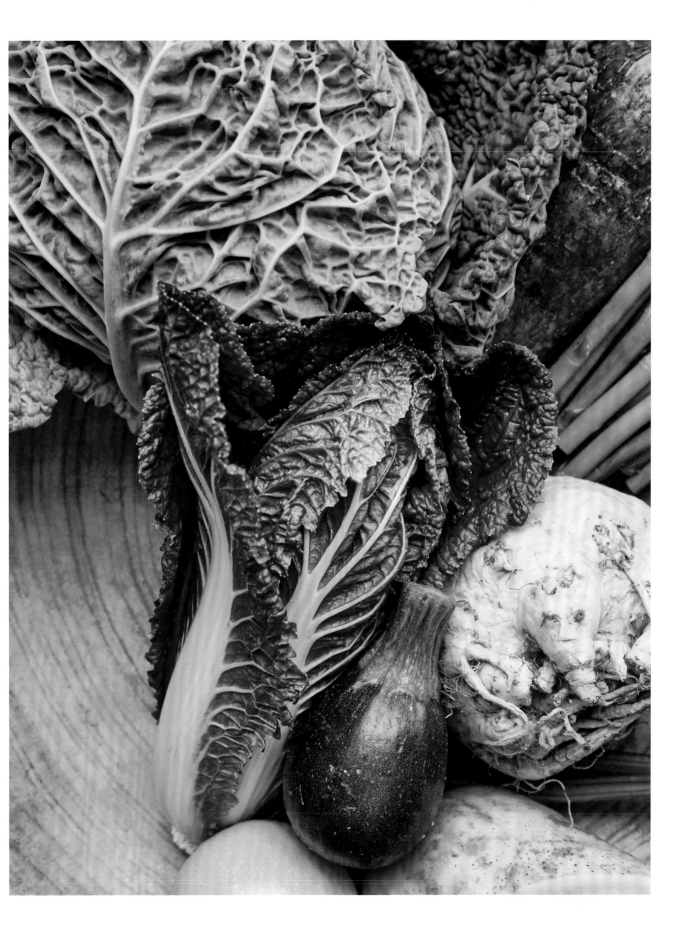

the meaning and purpose of food

I love food and I enjoy eating, but I stopped being a foodie. I no longer eat as a hobby or just for pleasure. If a dish is interesting and unusual yet it lacks nutrients or would be difficult to digest, I appreciate its originality but would not necessarily eat it. I also no longer direct my creativity toward transforming fruits and vegetables into unrecognizable—be they delicious—preparations only to show that it can be done.

I look at food as a source of deep nourishment, not entertainment. I gather the ingredients and recipes that deliver delightful flavors and textures naturally, without overly complicated preparation. If you are a person who enjoys cooking creatively but wants food to sustain your health, why not redirect your energy to learning what different ingredients can do *for you* rather than what else you can do *with them*? Instead of finding new ways to process or transform food externally, keep your cooking simple, and invest your time discovering how to support your body to best digest your meals and transform their nutrients and healing benefits into vitality. Do you lean toward fancy food for show or simple food for nourishment?

Ayurveda uses two main Sanskrit words to denote food: *anna* and *ahara*. *Anna* specifically relates to eatables in general, or the substances (i.e., micronutrients) that our bodies can easily assimilate and absorb. The salad you had yesterday will transform and become a part of your physical being within the next twenty-seven or so days, which is the time it takes for food to break down into smaller and smaller particles that can nourish each body tissue.

Ahara means "that which we take in," and it denotes not only food but anything else that we bring in through our senses—what we see, hear, smell, touch, or taste. Our body is a product of what we've taken in until now, especially from the food we've eaten. For example, if you have a problem with joints, pimples, or being overweight or underweight, these conditions are all a result of your past food choices. And the opposite is also true: your good health is a reward for eating good food in the right way, at the right time.

Make sure that your body recognizes the food you consume. The more that food's wholesomeness is denatured through processing, refining, or genetic modification, the less your physiology will recognize its molecules as something that are meant to be "taken in" and fully absorbed to provide deep tissue nourishment and mental satisfaction. The food substance that has not been absorbed begins to accumulate as semi-digested "sludge" that becomes a breeding ground for dis-ease. (I'll elaborate on this in the section on digestion, page 26).

In *The Way We Eat Now*, Bee Wilson speaks about "mismatches," or "the clashes between the new food reality and the persistence of human biology and culture adapted to earlier times." I find her words relevant to eating Ayurvedically as well—but this does not mean we must turn our clocks back in time and cook and eat exactly the way our ancestors or the authors of the ancient Ayurvedic texts did. That would be impossible because, as part of finding our balance, we need to adapt our way of eating to the modern realities of lifestyle, technology, and climate change. "Instead of looking backwards to some imagined past which we can never reclaim, we need to look forwards and have yet another change of taste," Wilson writes. To me, that change of taste is going back to accepting food as a source of nourishment by choosing wholesome, fresh, invigorating ingredients that our body can recognize and utilize completely.

The good news is that a vast variety of foods can give us both health and pleasure! My recipes in this book present ideas on how to accomplish that—they'll nourish your whole being while retaining your family's excitement at the table.

sensory perception of food's effects vs. nutrition facts

Ayurveda isn't so concerned about nutrition facts such as proteins, carbohydrates, and sugar, but instead investigates each ingredient's attributes to inform us what foods work for us as the unique individuals we are. While there's no debate that nutrition facts offer value, even more important is understanding how an ingredient interacts with and affects your individual health condition. Imagine that you and I ate a piece of cake of the exact same quality and quantity. We consumed the same number of calories and nutrients; however, our bodies responded differently— your piece of cake calmed your hunger and gave you energy, and mine gave me a dull sensation in my stomach and made me gain weight. Why? Each person's response to an ingredient is personal, and it depends on the person's digestive and metabolic strength. To determine which foods are most balancing for you, you first need to understand each ingredient's effects on human physiology.

In *What to Eat for How You Feel*, I detail the way Ayurveda describes each ingredient's attributes—its taste, qualities, metabolic effect, post-digestive effect, and healing properties. These attributes allow us to

interpret the energetics of food and how they affect us. In the recipe portion of this book, I profile featured ingredients according to these attributes. Knowing how ingredients act in your body and when to eat them will empower you to develop a deeper, more exciting connection with whole, plant-based foods. With such a connection, food will become poetry to you. It will heal and invigorate you. When you understand that cilantro pulls heavy metals from your body, you'll inherently feel more connected to cilantro. When you learn that kulthi lentils (a.k.a. horse gram) dissolve kidney stones and gallstones and any calcification in the body, you'll want to try them right away. And when you read that something as simple as toasted fennel seeds can relieve longstanding burning acidity in your stomach, you'll welcome fennel as a new friend.

When food lands on our tongue, we first experience its predominant taste—be it sweet, sour, salty, pungent, bitter, or astringent. Let us now explore the fascinating insights of how these tastes surpass what we feel on our palate and affect our physiology and mental capacity.

experiencing food through the six tastes

Ayurveda helps us deepen our perception and understanding of taste beyond what we experience with our tongue. Each taste of food can trigger a physiological, mental, and emotional response. While the emerging science of neurogastronomy continues to research our taste receptors, we can turn to the Ayurvedic texts that have described the attributes and effects of each of the six tastes.

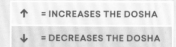

↑ = INCREASES THE DOSHA

↓ = DECREASES THE DOSHA

SWEET TASTE
Building & Nourishing Foods

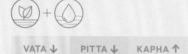

VATA ↓   PITTA ↓   KAPHA ↑

POSITIVE MENTAL RESPONSE: pleasure, satisfaction, joy, festivity

PHYSICAL RESPONSE: generates satiation, coats the mouth, soothes the sense organs, fulfills the cells' needs for growth and sustenance

FOOD EXAMPLES: rice and wheat, almonds and cashews, sweet potatoes and beets, milk and cream, meat (of course, all sweeteners are of predominant sweet taste)

It's important to understand that sweet taste does not necessarily mean sugary. Most foods that are heavier in nature, stabilizing, and nurturing are of sweet taste. Such foods build our body mass and enhance our strength and stamina.

Ayurveda recommends at least half of our meal to consist of building foods, and because these foods can be heavy, we use foods of the other five tastes to support the proper breakdown of these nurturing foods. However, eating foods of sweet taste in excess can cause the bitter results of weight gain, sluggishness, and mental fog.

SOUR TASTE
Digestive Foods

VATA ↓   PITTA ↑   KAPHA ↑

POSITIVE MENTAL RESPONSE: mental acuity, discernment, invigoration

PHYSICAL RESPONSE: increases salivation and hunger, enhances our ability to taste food better, cuts through heaviness

FOOD EXAMPLES: yogurt and aged cheese, vitamin C-rich citrus and pineapple, vinegar and fermented foods

Foods of sour taste are light to digest, stimulate the appetite, clear the taste buds, and protect fats in the body from going rancid. Sour foods in excess can create acidity, heartburn, skin issues, premature aging, or an overly critical mind.

Acidic foods are meant to be served in small quantities or as a side dish, such as a pickle, a sauce, or a fruit snack. I often garnish dishes with a little lime juice as a taste enhancer.

SALTY TASTE
Flavor-Enhancing Foods

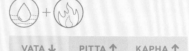

VATA ↓   PITTA ↑   KAPHA ↑

POSITIVE MENTAL RESPONSE: mental ease, desire, zest for life

PHYSICAL RESPONSE: cuts through tissue membranes and draws out water

FOOD EXAMPLES: different types of salt (sea, rock, black), different types of seaweed (kombu, kelp, dulse), seafood

Salt relieves obstructions in the body channels. In excess, salty foods can cause high blood pressure, skin dryness or rashes, hair loss, accelerated aging, water retention, eye problems, and more.

Salt brings forth the other five tastes, and this is why when a dish lacks salt, we find it bland.

PUNGENT TASTE
Sharp & Stimulating Foods

VATA ↑	PITTA ↑	KAPHA ↓

POSITIVE MENTAL RESPONSE: ambition, motivation

PHYSICAL RESPONSE: stimulates a sharp and penetrating transportation of nutrients, creates heat and dryness

FOOD EXAMPLES: chiles, onion and garlic, horseradish and mustard greens, cloves and mustard seeds

Pungent foods heat up the body, create a sense of lightness, and improve our digestive capacity. Pungents spark our metabolism, assist in weight loss, open the circulatory channels, clear phlegm and fungus, prevent blood clotting, kill microbes, and give our skin a glow. A recent study suggests that people who regularly eat pungent foods live longer!

It can be tempting to consume a lot of pungent foods because they are so bold and charging. However, too much pungency can lead to increased dryness in the lining of the digestive tract and body tissues, colitis, ulcers, diarrhea, redness of the skin, broken capillaries, irritability, and even aggression. Uncontrolled, explosive anger is the most destructive emotion, and it can lead to chronic inflammation. If you're experiencing any of these issues, decrease your intake of pungent foods.

BITTER TASTE
Cleansing Foods

VATA ↑	PITTA ↓	KAPHA ↓

POSITIVE MENTAL RESPONSE: clarity, mental focus, desire for change, insightfulness

PHYSICAL RESPONSE: dries up moisture, reduces body bulk (tissues), creates coolness and lightness

FOOD EXAMPLES: broccoli rabe and kale, bitter melon and dandelion greens, coffee and chocolate, burdock root and turmeric

Bitter-tasting foods increase alkalinity and eliminate acidic toxins, draw out worms and parasites, cleanse the mouth and clear the throat, detoxify the liver and the blood, flush the lymphatic system, reduce sugar cravings, and lower high blood sugar. I always think of bitter as the taste that lets me enjoy sweetness.

Prepare bitter foods as a side dish. They can be an excellent digestive when taken at the beginning of your meal. Too much bitter taste can cause depletion and dryness in the body, anemia, low blood pressure, constipation, vertigo, premature wrinkles, dissatisfaction, self-doubt, and other bitter emotions.

ASTRINGENT TASTE
Moisture-Absorbing Foods

VATA ↑	PITTA ↓	KAPHA ↓

POSITIVE MENTAL RESPONSE: optimism, well-being, introspection

PHYSICAL RESPONSE: pulls in moisture from the mouth and tissues, causing a puckering reaction, creates dryness

FOOD EXAMPLES: pomegranate and unripe banana, spinach and asparagus, lentils and beans, black or green tea and nicotine, nutmeg

The astringent-tasting foods lighten the body, clear the tongue, help with absorption of nutrients, purify the blood, decrease fat tissues, and stop diarrhea. In excess, astringent foods can slow digestion, cause gas, constipation, cramps, and unhealthy thirst. They will also make your mind susceptible to fear, insecurity, or self-absorption.

I prepare astringent foods in combination with water or fat to reduce their drying effect. Ayurveda recommends we end each meal with an astringent substance, such as a tiny spoon of honey or a small cup of buttermilk, to tell the body "This concludes my eating." (See also End-of-Meal Astringents on page 235.) You'd be surprised how effective this is in preventing you from overeating!

When preparing a balancing meal, think about how you can incorporate foods of all six tastes but in the proportions relevant to the seasonal balance of your doshas:

SWEET, SOUR, SALTY: Use them more in late fall and winter and when your Vata is high.

SWEET, BITTER, ASTRINGENT: Use them more in summer and early fall and when your Pitta is high.

PUNGENT, BITTER, ASTRINGENT: Use them more in late winter and spring and when your Kapha is high or when you're detoxing.

digestion: your precedent for good or bad health

In my late twenties and thirties, I was a victim of chronic digestive issues. I kept eliminating foods from my diet to a point when there was hardly anything left on my OK list, and food turned from a source of enjoyment to cries of misery. I was always tired after eating lunch, not realizing that my digestive weakness was the beginning of a bigger problem, an auto-immune disorder. Thanks to my Ayurvedic healers, I learned that the solution was not to limit the foods I was eating but to fix my digestion.

If there is one aspect of human physiology that everyone should learn about, I'd say it is digestion. Ayurveda considers it the most essential process in our body because it sets the stage for either consistent good health or sickness from many of the diseases we experience today.

Anything that we ingest, including food, liquids, herbs, medications, viruses, and environmental pollutants, must go through this process. When in good working order, the digestion process extracts macronutrients and micronutrients from what we take in and eliminates the unwanted wastes, pathogens, and so on.

Ayurveda identifies the "cooking" or transformative power of digestion with the term *agni*. It can literally mean "fire," but it denotes more of a process than an element or thing. The digestive *agni* in our body is the microrepresentation of the cosmic *agni*, one of the components of *prana* that I explained above. I like Dr. Bhaswati Bhattacharya's translation of *agni*: "that which engulfs a substance and transforms it into another." In modern medicine, *agni* is known as the enzymatic function that participates in all digestive and cellular processes, transforming nutrients and making them easy to assimilate. *Agni* is our capacity to metabolize—not only food into energy but *ahara* in general, or that which we consume with all our senses. When *agni* is too low or too high, your metabolism will experience its corresponding effects. For example, if the *agni* transforming your fat tissue is weak, you could experience an overaccumulation of fat; you may feel a lack of confidence and low energy. If your *agni* is too high, your hyper-metabolism could lead to drastic weight loss; you won't be able to deeply integrate your life experiences. Ayurveda identifies thirteen types of *agni* that moderate the transformation processes in the body and mind. The initial one is encountered in the stomach and duodenum, and it governs our ability to digest food. Its function has a ripple effect on all other metabolic processes in the body or the mind, including our ability to digest life as we experience it through our thoughts, emotions, and ideas.

The three doshas control and modify *agni*. When our doshas are functioning well, we will have pleasant *agni* and enjoy good digestion and energy. When Pitta is too high, it's like excessive "fuel" for a fire, making it blaze too strongly. In the body, this is exemplified by of hypermetabolism leading to a "fiery" digestive imbalance that "burns" the food's nutrients before you can fully assimilate them.

When Kapha is too high, it's like having too much moisture around a fire—it dampens and lowers the flame. This will diminish the production of stomach acid and weaken your *agni*; you will experience the "earthy" type of digestion, which is sluggish and heavy.

When Vata is too high, it's like a fan blowing into a fire—the flames waver, appearing unstable and irregular. In the body, this translates to an erratic *agni*, sometimes too high and sometimes too low. It creates the "airy" type of digestion, which manifests as a variable appetite, gas, and bloating.

your diet and your immunity

Today, digestive problems predominate more than ever before. Incomplete digestion and poor assimilation of nutrients have become the new normal—so much so that we often don't even notice them until they really disturb us. I think a major reason for these massive digestive disorders is the infiltration of ultra-processed, high-calorie/low-nutrient foods since the 1960s, including refined and artificial sweeteners and vegetable oils, chips, soda, cookies, candy, ice cream, processed breakfast cereals, burgers, fries, fake meat— what future do they summon for us? I can't overestimate the importance of consuming wholesome, recognizable, bioavailable foods to maintain strong *agni* and longevity.

The tragic consequences of the global coronavirus pandemic had a silver lining: many of us became more concerned about eating and living healthier. Adopting a healthier diet and lifestyle calls for quitting immune-compromising, clogging, and processed foods and choosing to focus on self-care through nutrition and disease prevention.

Ayurveda is very clear that there is a direct relationship between the health of our gut and the strength of our immune system. Earlier we discussed the function of *agni*, or digestive and metabolic fire. It helps not only to digest food but it also plays a protective role in our overall immunity. *Agni* is designed to discriminate between nutritive and toxic substances as well as pathogens such as viruses, bacteria, and parasites. A strong *agni* can "burn up" unwanted microorganisms and pollutants as necessary. It can also tackle the common gut irritants: oxalates, gluten, lactose, and lectins. *Agni* is our first line of immunity, and when it diminishes, we become more susceptible to disease.

To maintain good health, keep your *agni* appropriately stoked and regulated. Ayurveda advises us to learn how to assess the state of our *agni* and digestion and select our balancing foods accordingly. Please note that even though the doshas control *agni*, your constitution does not determine the foods you need to eat for the rest of your life. Your *agni* will fluctuate based on the dosha that is currently out of balance; therefore, you need to select the foods for the strength of your *agni* and the dosha that needs correction. Refer to the Digestion Questionnaire (page 249) to assess which type of digestion you're currently experiencing.

Your body will reciprocate your efforts to be healthy. When you nourish yourself wholesomely and maintain an optimum *agni*, you will build a lasting vitality that Ayurveda calls *ojas*. *Ojas* is your reward for maintaining good digestion; it is the essence of all transformations in the body. After you've eaten and properly digested, assimilated, and absorbed the food's nutrients into your every cell, the final and most precious extract produced by your body is *ojas*. Strong *ojas* gives a glow to your skin and eyes, ensures a strong stamina and immunity, and helps you respond to stress with ease. If you experience these positive symptoms, you're taking care of your health properly.

Now, what happens to the food particles that we do not assimilate? Where do they go?

semi-digested food:
the root cause of inflammation

In the best health scenario, the food you eat is completely engulfed by *agni*, and your digestive system grabs what's useful and sends it into the body tissues and drives what's not useful out for elimination. If, however, your *agni* is low, undigested protein and fat molecules can't be fully absorbed, and they will linger in the small intestine, irritating it and causing allergies to heavy foods, such as those containing gluten, lectins, or lactose. These unused food particles will end up in the lymphatic system, which also acts as one of the "garbage disposals" in the body. In time, the lymphatic "drains" can become clogged. A congested lymphatic system can lead to the accumulation of fatigue, belly fat, bloat, brain fog, and more. Ayurveda calls this semi-digested, "unripe" food residue *ama*. It is the food that we've eaten but has not transformed to become a part of our body.

There is a bidirectional correlation between the state of *agni* and the accumulation of ama: less *agni* leads to more *ama*. The more that *ama* accumulates and clogs the pathways in our body, the weaker our *agni* becomes. *Ama* is heavy and sticky; it attaches to the coronary arteries, digestive tract, lungs, sinuses, and brain, and thus becomes the main cause of inflammation. This does not happen overnight—it is the result of years of eating unsuitable foods.

Please note that there is a difference between building the bulk of your body (e.g., gaining weight by building muscle) and building *ama*. Ayurveda views the cause of obesity to be not overnourishment but the kind of depleted *agni* that leads to an accumulation and stagnation of *ama*, which makes us gain weight.

Even though the body does not make a chemical connection with *ama*, our

Some Characteristics and Symptoms of *Ama* and *Ama-visha*

	Characteristics	Symptoms
Ama	Cold, sticky, slow-moving	Fatigue, congestion, heaviness, coated tongue, bad breath
Ama-visha	Hot, sharp, acidic, fast-moving	Inflammation, pain, chronic diseases, autoimmune issues, terminal illness

physiology has a natural ability to eliminate it. However, if our challenged *agni* continuously struggles to keep up with our unhealthy eating habits, *ama* begins to pile up in the intestinal tract and turns into an acidic, fermented residue called *ama-visha*. Eventually, *ama* and *ama-visha* will end up in the bloodstream and circulate within the body, searching for its weakest spots to settle. This is how semi-digested food gradually inhibits our body functions and leads to chronic inflammation and disease.

Because *ama* and *ama-visha* have different characteristics, their purging requires specific and contrasting treatment protocols. Please consult with an Ayurvedic doctor for the approach best suited for you.

Here are the five most common eating and lifestyle habits that perpetuate the *agni-ama* cycle:

1. Not eating food when you're hungry (skipping or delaying meals)

2. Overeating: continuing to eat even though you're full or eating anything before your previous meal has been fully digested (for a healthy person, it usually takes about four hours to digest a full meal)

3. Eating a meal of foods that don't digest well together (see Ayurvedic Food Compatibility Chart on page 244)

4. Being in a negative state of mind: dwelling in excessive anxiety, fear, anger, frustration, sadness, loneliness

5. Having poor quality sleep: going to bed late (after 10 p.m.), frequently waking up at night, not sleeping enough

If you are looking for ways to reset your organism and live healthier, I'd suggest you start improving on the areas listed in these five points. You'd be surprised how even small adjustments in these areas will give you quick results.

In *What to Eat for How You Feel*, I explain the different types of digestion and how to balance each one with foods and spices. In this book, I will focus on the digestibility of featured ingredients and how to incorporate them into recipes.

food suitability

I hope that by now you're beginning to understand the importance of eating food for balance, which will help you experience the joy of maintaining good health. Now, let's discuss how to select your balancing foods. I am not going to give you a list of dosha balancing ingredients and tell you what you should eat. Rather, I will help you understand the principles behind using food for balance and nourishment so that you can make the right decision for yourself or others in any given circumstance. It all boils down to whether your choice of food is suitable or unsuitable for your current situation.

Ayurveda describes eighteen categories of food compatibility, and the most important of them are suitability in terms of your

- state of digestion/strength of *agni*,

- health condition,

- dosha-balancing needs,

- climate and geographical location,

- time of day, season, and life (age),

- physical activity, and

- upbringing.

First check in with yourself and see how you're feeling: How does your stomach feel—acidic or bloated or heavy, or are you simply hungry? Depending on what your stomach is telling you, select foods that have opposing qualities. For example, if you're experiencing heartburn or acidity, you're likely also feeling hot or sharp in some way. So, to counteract these sensations, favor soothing and calming foods that are predominantly sweet, bitter, and astringent in taste (Pitta-reducing), such as rice, leafy greens, or mung dal; avoid foods that are sour and pungent (Pitta-aggravating), such as fermented items and chile peppers, and decrease your salt intake.

How hungry are you? The hungrier you are, the higher your *agni* is, and the easier it will be for you to digest heavier foods or eat a larger portion. If you're not hungry, either fast until you are or drink a digestive tea with ginger to spark your appetite.

Health conditions (including environmental or food allergies) will limit your dietary choices. As for your dosha-balancing needs, select foods with opposing attributes of the dosha that feels too high for you. For example, if your Vata is high and you're feeling cold and ungrounded, have a warm and nourishing stew, such as my Minestrone (page 51). If your Pitta needs correction and you're feeling heated or agitated, favor a calming meal of Plain Basmati Rice (page 64) and Summer Curry (page 128). If your unbalanced Kapha is making you feel sluggish and in need of lightening up, try the Braised Purple Cabbage (page 117). Consult with the Seasonal Recipe Guide on page 242 for more meal ideas.

It is best, but not always possible, to eat all locally grown and seasonal ingredients. The food that grows in the same water, air, and sunshine that you are exposed to will metabolize best for you. However, in most parts of the world, it is difficult to use 100 percent locally grown ingredients. I live in New York City and use mung dal and spices from India, limes and avocados from California, and wild rice from Canada. However, I buy most of my fresh fruits and vegetables from our local farmers market. To appease my quest for locally grown, during the warm season, I grow eighteen culinary herbs on my balcony!

Time of day is also important, as the strength of our *agni* varies with our circadian rhythms. Enjoy heavier, bigger meal portions between ten in the morning and two in the afternoon, keep dinner light, and don't eat too late at night unless you're very hungry. If you're hungry late at night, keep your meal light and free from very pungent or acidic foods, which are stimulating, making it more difficult to fall asleep.

The level of your physical activity is reflected in your metabolism: the more physically active you are, the more energy you burn, and thus the more building foods—those that have a predominant sweet taste—and larger portions you need.

And finally, all of us grow up accustomed to eating a specific cuisine—these are our comfort foods, and our body is habituated to digesting them, even if they are incompatible according to Ayurveda. For example, growing up in Bulgaria, I ate a lot of cheese with bread. Cheese and wheat is a heavy combination, but because my body has been familiar with it since childhood, I can digest them well today. However, I struggle to digest glass noodles and tempeh because they were not part of my upbringing, and I am not accustomed to eating them as an adult. Some people thrive on rice but struggle with digesting wheat; some can't give up eating meat because it is so genetically encoded in their body. Think of the foods that were a regular part of your diet since childhood—these are likely your comfort foods that you probably gravitate to when you're stressed out. Are you able to digest them well as an adult?

Your comfort foods may not always be the foods that are good and balancing for your current situation, though. If you grew up eating a lot of junk food, don't use it as an excuse for your poor diet today. In adulthood, it takes your body about three months to become acquainted with a new ingredient.

To upgrade your comfort foods, you could create the fresh, wholesome versions of the quick pleasers you indulged in as a child. In this book, I give you delicious recipes for some comfort foods like pizza, chocolate chip cookies, and sesame crackers that will hopefully satisfy your childhood craving and leave you feeling balanced. Another way to make your comfort foods more digestible is to cook them with more spices and herbs. My recipes will give you ideas on how to do that.

your meal portions

I was raised in a culture that posed a lot of restrictions—on self-expression, connections to the world, and food variety. My family never starved, but our food choices were limited. I was taught to finish all the food on my plate, even if I was past my point of fullness. For many years of my adult life, I followed the same pattern—I ate all the food in front of me to avoid feeling the guilt often associated with "wasting" any of it. My perception of deprivation led me to eat too much. But I wondered, How is feeding my body more than it needs a good thing? Isn't *that* a waste of food? Isn't it more beneficial and kinder to give away or compost the extra food than it is to eat it? When I eat more than I need, I'm really just abusing my body by putting on extra weight or developing digestive problems.

Many people today experience the opposite of my childhood circumstance: they have an abundance of food, and thus they overeat simply because they can or because they need to fill a void. Food addictions can spring from either deprivation or abundance, but in both cases the result will be the loss of joy and pleasure in tasting; food becomes a source of anxiety. This can be exacerbated by

the memory of emotional attachments and physical traumas related to food that many of us carry. Only by healing these traumas can we create more space for joy and pleasure. If you're a parent, be mindful of the food memories you're generating in your children.

Another way to lose your appreciation of food is by misunderstanding what it means to cut back and thus not eating enough. This is the opposite of indulgence. I lived in yoga ashrams in Europe and India for fifteen years. Simple living strengthened my mind and character, helped me treasure time, and directed my activities toward self-improvement and service to others. I would never give back these years. However, in my neophyte zealotry to give up material entanglement, I also "desensitized" myself and lost my ability to experience and process joy, including enjoyment from food, because I did not want to glut in false pleasures. My understanding of the intent behind detachment was distorted: I thought that suffering was a sacred act. By depriving myself of joy and pleasure, I was not fully present in my life, and I justified my detachment with my deepening spirituality.

Maturing emotionally and spiritually helped me discern between false pleasure that's attached to addiction and true pleasure that leads to unity, a surrender to spirit, and service. Connecting with the divine source of pleasure is so liberating! After all, a spiritual practice is meant to make us jolly, not grumpy. Once I gave myself permission to let joy and pleasure rewire me, I had to learn how to internalize them. I started enjoying food again, but it took a higher level of consciousness to get there, and eventually I happily felt a strong spiritual connection to my food and eating patterns. As you metabolize pleasure, it ripples out to the world as an invitation for others to have joy. On the contrary, if you live in denial of joy, you will emit gloom and deprivation.

Eating with self-awareness can strengthen your digestion and immune system. It can also protect you from overeating because its inherent slow pace (about twenty to thirty minutes per meal) allows you to listen to your body's wisdom and stop eating when it says, "Hey, we've had enough." Learning how to metabolize the joy and pleasure of eating will help you eat less and enjoy more.

HOW TO DETERMINE YOUR MEAL PORTION

The first step to quit overeating is to know your threshold of fullness. Even though our stomach capacity is unique to each of us, Ayurveda makes it easy to determine. If you're in good health, by the end of your meal, your stomach should be

- half-full with solid food,

- a quarter-full with liquid (from a drink, water, or soup, for example), and

- a quarter empty.

mindful practice

I make time to eat. I present myself with gratitude to the food in front of me and I slow down to chew each bite in silence, noticing the tastes and flavors that unfold in my mouth. When I get a nice feeling, I let my body and mind pause and revel in pleasure: "Wow, this tastes amazing!" Feeling joy with each bite, I connect the beauty of the plant or herb with spirit and I take that in. This fills my heart with gratitude for the gift of food.

Fullness does not mean stuffed: it means full enough, content. You will feel satisfied but not heavy. This is the time to stop eating, even if you still have food on your plate. Leaving that quarter portion of your stomach empty provides space for the food to "churn" and transform into a nutritive juice that moves down your digestive tract in a timely manner.

The opposite of overeating can also be harmful to your health. I'm not talking about skipping a meal here or there but rather not eating enough in one sitting. When more than one-quarter of your stomach is empty after eating your meal, then your meal portion is insufficient. This, too, will distort your doshas and *agni*, leaving you hungry, dissatisfied, and unable to concentrate. There is a saying in Ayurveda that if the body tissues are not adequately fed, they will start to eat themselves by drawing from their reserves and gradually deplete the whole organism. Starving the body is not the answer. If you're trying to lose weight, try the Ayurvedic approach to eating rather than restricting the amount of food you eat.

Ayurveda does not advise determining your proper meal portion using a calorie or weight measurement. Instead, it is recommended to use a personalized unit of measurement called an *anjali*, which is equivalent to the quantity that you can fill in the space formed from joining your two palms together like a bowl. Two *anjalis* is the recommended amount of food per meal, and everyone's *anjali* is different. A child's *anjali*, for example, will be smaller in volume than an adult's *anjali*. Your meal portion also depends on your current appetite, the time of day, or your health condition.

I've noticed that people in the US often don't appreciate the value of food beyond its price or connect meal size with the nutrition it provides. A smaller portion of nutrient-dense food will satiate you faster and nourish you deeper compared to a larger volume of ultra-processed fast food. Portion and price also tend to clash: you can purchase a large burger, fries, and a twenty-four-ounce soda for a fraction of the price of a smaller portion of a fresh, wholesome meal prepared with vegetables, lentils, or grains. A five-scoop serving of ice cream loaded with unrecognizable substances costs as much as one scoop of a frozen delight made with four real ingredients. Could ill health be the long-term cost of eating cheap convenience meals prepared from frozen and canned goods? I think so.

Ayurveda considers food healing not only when it is selected and prepared properly but also when it is served in the right amount. A scoop of ice cream could be healing for someone with high stomach acid—its heavy and cooling qualities will offer immediate relief. Five scoops, however, would be *ama*-producing. If you eat too much—even of your most balancing foods—you will feel fatigued or get a stomachache. The three-quarter-full principle is essential to feeling energized. After all, eating is a sacred act of bringing energy, not calories, into your body.

When at home, try eating with the tips of your fingers, without utensils. It might seem uncultured and messy to you, but try it at least for fun. With practice, you'll appreciate how eating this way engages many of your senses and enhances your relationship to food. This ultimately benefits your digestion because the direct connection between your sense organs sends a signal to your brain to release the exact amount of necessary digestive enzymes. Additionally, eating with your fingers perfectly portions each morsel by allowing you to only pick up as much as your finger grab can hold—this will help you chew better. You'd be surprised how well this style of eating will lead to contentment with less food!

mindful practice

Sit on a chair or cross-legged on the floor and look at the food you're about to eat. Move your face toward the dish and smell it. Then use your fingers on your right hand to touch it, feel its temperature and texture, and then use your fingers to put it in your mouth. Chew that morsel until it has liquified, swallow with pleasure, and repeat with another bite. At the end of your meal, remain seated for a couple of minutes and express gratitude: "I have enough. I am satisfied and content. I am grateful."

BEWARE OF CLOGGING FOODS

Earlier we discussed how balanced health stems from an optimal flow of *prana*, meaning there are no obstructions or "traffic jams" in the physical and energetic pathways. We also learned that *ama* (semi-digested food) or *ama-visha* (fermented *ama*) is the substance that blocks the channels.

Our body consists of thousands of channels that transport and deliver nutrients, fluids, and even subtle vibrations of energy from one area of the body to another. Both macrochannels and microchannels are the pathways that facilitate all circulation in the body. Some examples include the digestive tract, sinuses, ear canals, and blood vessels. Think of these channels in your body as the pipes in your house. And just like pipes, your body's channels can get clogged. That would be a problem, wouldn't it?

The clogging buildup happens gradually, usually starting in the microchannels—that's why we may not notice it for quite some time. Most people experience its effects with the drastic hormonal changes in middle age. For women, the more clogging there is in your body, the more challenging menopause will be.

Clogging foods are those that are heavy for the average person to digest. One consequence of eating these types of foods is their tendency to thicken the bile, which is

essential for breaking down fats—not only from food but also from fat-soluble toxins and fatty hormones (e.g., estrogen). When we consistently eat fatty, hard-to-digest foods, the gallbladder becomes sluggish and challenged with thickened bile, gallstones, gallbladder inflammation, and other issues.

Here is a list of common channel-clogging and bile-thickening foods, which I recommend avoiding or using rarely, in small amounts, in order to keep your "pipes" clear:

- frozen/ice-cold foods and beverages

- deep-fried foods

- hard-to-digest oils and oil supplements: vegetable oils, hydrogenated fats and margarines, fish oil, flax seed oil, and other oils rich in omega-3s, etc.

- cold dairy—especially Greek yogurt, cold milk, ice cream, frozen yogurt

- aged cheeses (typically the hard cheeses)

- leftovers

- chocolate

- nut butters

- red meats

- sheep's milk

- refined flours and sugars

foods for daily consumption vs. medicinal foods for occasional use

Ayurveda classifies food in yet another way: for daily consumption and for occasional medicinal use. Both are healing and nurturing, but their application is different.

Foods for daily consumption are meant for nourishment—they build the bulk tissues in our body and give us energy and strength. We can eat them regularly in larger amounts with hardly any unintended effects. When preparing a nourishing meal, consider the proportions of the six tastes from largest to smallest quantity in this order: sweet, sour, salty, pungent, bitter, astringent.

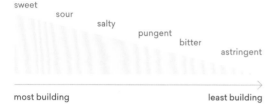

Medicinal foods can be very potent and with strong effects. They have the capacity to heal profoundly and are meant to be prescribed as medicine: in small amounts, periodically, and only when you need their help to correct an imbalance. When using medicinal ingredients in meals for treatment, consider the proportions of the six tastes from largest to smallest quantity in this order: astringent, bitter, pungent, salty, sour, sweet.

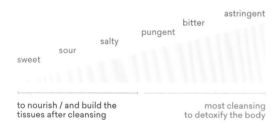

Flax seeds are an example of a medicinal food. They are high in omega-3 fatty acids and serve as a prebiotic, but they are quite heating for the liver and possibly too heavy for your body to digest fully. An overconsumption of flax can lead to problems with the eyes, liver, and reproductive fluid. Ayurvedic doctors prescribe flax for certain Vata and Kapha disorders, for a short amount of time.

Spices are kind of in between—they are the bridge between food and medicine and are to be used in small amounts in both daily meals and in herbal supplements.

Here are a few examples of foods in each category, according to the Shaka Vansiya lineage:

Foods for Daily Consumption	Medicinal Foods for Occasional Use
Rice	Moringa
Wheat	Onion
Quinoa	Garlic
Dairy	Flax
Most vegetables	Bitter melon
Most Fruits	Amla (fruit)
Nuts and seeds	Medicinal herbs
Ghee, olive oil, coconut oil	Bone broth
	Mushrooms
Unrefined sweeteners	

Food and our interaction with it have the power to create *or* eliminate physical blockages and mental suppression, support *or* distort our flow of *prana*, and shorten *or* prolong our life. In the following pages I will help you deepen your food wisdom by learning in depth about ingredients from both the daily consumption and medicinal categories. By using these ingredients in my delicious and easy-to-digest recipes, you can take care of your health right there in your kitchen!

Before we begin cooking, let's step into your cooking space and look at the tools and equipment you'll need to make your Ayurvedic meal preparation efficient and joyful.

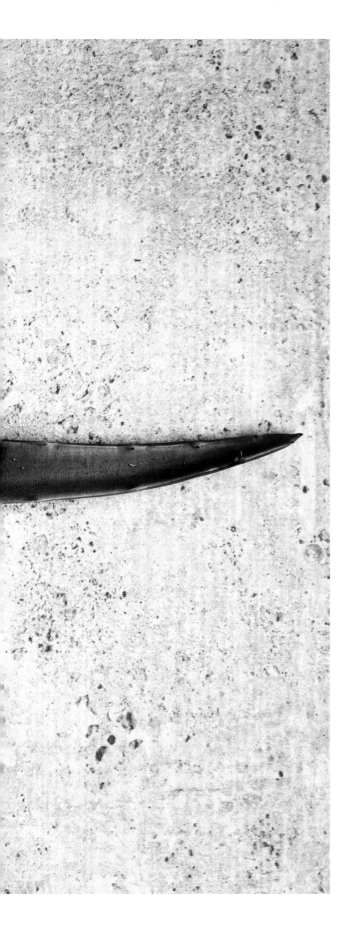

a
modern
guide
to
ayurvedic
home
cooking

kitchen setup and tools

I love being in the kitchen. I often spend more time in it than planned. Having lived in apartments and houses of different sizes, I have cooked in just about every possible kitchen setting—from a kitchenette with a stove, tiny sink, and a one-square-foot countertop to a spacious room with natural light and all the cabinet and countertop space that I ever dreamt of. Whatever your current kitchen setting is, arrange it as your place of joy and excitement, and organize it according to your personal cooking style. Whenever I am setting up or reorganizing my kitchen, I use these words to guide me in the process: comfortable, clean, efficient, and inspiring.

As you prepare and cook your food, ask yourself: "Do I flow in this kitchen?" If you are constantly moving an item out of your way or are bumping into something, this is a sign that it's not in the right place, and you should store it somewhere else, or consider giving it a new home. Which cabinet is the most comfortable for you to access your spices and oils? Which countertop is convenient for assembling the ingredients? Are your cutting board and knives on or near this countertop? Store your cookware according to frequency of use—the pots and pans you use most often are best stored in the front. The same principle applies to your dry pantry—situate the ingredients you use most frequently in the front of the shelf. For best preservation, store all ingredients in airtight, labeled containers in a dark and dry place. Give away the equipment or ingredients you never use. Initially, this may be hard to do, but I believe once you do it, you'll discover a new and exhilarating space.

Just like we favor high-quality ingredients, it is equally important to select healthy and nontoxic cookware over the unhealthy or chemically reactive ones. A nourishing stew made of the best ingredients but cooked and stirred in an aluminum pot will probably leave traces of the pot's heavy metal (aluminum) in your system. In Ayurvedic cooking, not only do we always think about what and how to cook but also the material of the cookware— all of these practices will affect the medicinal properties of the food.

HEALTHY COOKWARE IS MADE FROM

- high-quality stainless steel,
- lead-free clay,
- glass,
- seasoned cast iron,
- stone,
- ceramic,
- unchipped enamel, or
- food-grade silicone.

UNHEALTHY COOKWARE IS MADE FROM

- aluminum,
- chemical nonstick surfaces,
- lead-containing clay pots,
- plastic,
- rusty iron, or
- materials that mimic ceramic.

SIZE

For your pot and pan inventory, consider the number of people you typically cook for and make that your baseline. If at any point you need to cook for more or fewer people, adjust the cookware size accordingly.

1 TO 2 PEOPLE

- two 1½- to 3-quart pots
- two 8- to 10-inch sauté pans and/or skillets

3 TO 4 PEOPLE

- two 3- to 6-quart pots
- two 8- to 12-inch sauté pans and/or skillets

5 TO 8 PEOPLE

- three 6- to 10-quart pots
- one 12-inch (or larger) sauté pan and/or skillet or two 8- to 10-inch sauté pans and/or skillets

KITCHEN TOOLS

Here are the essential tools you will need for preparing the recipes in this book.

CUTTING/SLICING/CRUSHING

- chef's knife
- paring knife
- serrated knife
- wooden cutting board
- bench scraper
- grater
- peeler
- mandoline slicer
- mortar and pestle

MEASURING

- set of stainless steel measuring spoons
- set of stainless steel measuring cups
- 4-cup measuring cup for liquids
- chef's thermometer (33–200°F)
- kitchen scale

COOKING

- 1½-quart saucepan with lid
- two 3- to 4-quart saucepans with lids
- 10- to 12-inch heavy sauté pan with lid
- well-seasoned 10-inch cast-iron griddle
- one or two baking sheets: 9 x 13 inches, 13 x 18 inches
- baking dishes: cake pan, 8 x 8-inch dish
- steamer or steaming basket
- three mixing bowls: small, medium, large (stainless steel or glass)
- two or three mixing and serving spoons (wooden and stainless steel)
- soup ladle
- spatulas (silicone, wooden, and stainless steel)
- two-pronged fork (for fluffing grains)

STRAINING

- set of fine-mesh strainers (small, medium, large)
- colander
- cheesecloth (ideally unbleached)
- nut milk bag

ELECTRIC APPLIANCES

These recommended appliances are for small-scale home cooking. Select the size that is most appropriate for you and your family's needs.

- spice or coffee grinder (to grind spices and nuts)
- blender (to finely puree soups, desserts, and drinks; to make nut milks)
- food processor (to save time and energy chopping, grinding, and grating)
- Instant Pot (to make yogurt, slow cook, and keep food warm)
- grain mill (if you bake frequently)

about the ingredients I use

As an Ayurvedic chef, high-quality ingredients are top priority for me because they are much more likely to deliver all of the desirable healing benefits that they boast. Although some of these ingredients can be more expensive than their inferior counterparts (depending on your location and the time of year), I prioritize them over spending money on gambling, alcohol, drugs, and excessive pleasures so I can provide my family with delicious and healing food. Budget your food costs according to your financial capacity. Keep in mind that purchasing dried beans and cooking them fresh is more economical than buying canned beans. Cooking at home is less expensive than eating out. Growing herbs in your garden is cheaper than buying them in bunches. How can you restructure your cooking and eating patterns to free up some money so that you can increase the variety and quality of fresh fruits, vegetables, lentils, and grains in your daily meals?

You may notice that I adopt some less-known ingredients. They may be uncommon in one region and easily available in another. My readers live all over the world, hence the wide variety of ingredients in my recipes. As a country of world immigrants, the US hosts every possible cuisine on earth. I am fortunate as a New Yorker because I find it easy to source international ingredients: I can purchase fresh sweet tamarind, taro root, chana dal, einkorn flour, kulthi lentils, and green chiles from a couple of grocery stores just around the corner from where I live. If you don't have this advantage and are curious to try a hard-to-find ingredient, search for it online. If that fails, then either omit it or try to replace it with an item of similar taste and texture. For example, in place of einkorn flour, try spelt four, or in place of taro root, try yucca root.

Diversifying your diet with these "new" ingredients will bring you a multitude of nutrients and health benefits. I imagine you'll be pleasantly surprised with the deliciousness and nourishment that you'll create from them, so I encourage you to explore and expand your pantry. The Sourcing section in the ingredient profiles and the Glossary (page 246) are additional helpful tools for learning more about where to purchase foods.

SALT: I used Soma Salt (a.k.a. saindhava) while creating all recipes. Soma Salt is a little less salty than other types of salt, so if you're using sea salt, kosher salt, or Himalayan salt, reduce the salt amount by a pinch or two.

OLIVE OIL: I use high-quality extra virgin olive oil (see Sources, page 248)

GHEE: I use Divya's Ayurvedic Cultured Ghee (see Sources, page 248)

ASAFOETIDA: I use The Best Hing Ever by Pure Indian Foods (see Sources, page 248). This is a pure and very strong asafoetida, which is why I add only a tiny pinch to a dish. Increase the amount if you're using the common asafoetida sold in Indian grocery stores (which I don't recommend because it's mixed with unwanted substances).

MILK: I use raw or pasteurized organic, non-homogenized milk from grass-fed cows.

FLOUR: I use freshly milled flours, often sifted. Packaged flour is more compact and of different volume measurement than sifted flour. For best results, follow the weight instead of cup measurements.

time-saving tips for preparing fresh meals daily

My friend Michael Halsband is not only an extraordinary photographer—he's one of the most committed yoga practitioners and home cooks I've met. I asked him, "How do you manage to cook every day, considering your unpredictable schedule as an artist?" His reply was, "I practice yoga and cooking as an investment into my well-being. Many people use the 'I don't have time' excuse to not do the things that are good for them while wasting time on things that don't matter as much. If you spend less time browsing the internet and instead do much more rewarding activities like yoga and cooking for yourself and your family, you will still have plenty of time for all the time-wasting stuff we all do. The method of yoga and cooking and living the Ayurvedic way helps me to take care of myself, and then, as a result, my mind and heart naturally turn outward to take care of others—this completes the circle of universal love." I appreciate Michael's mindset: taking the time to cook fresh meals is time invested, not time wasted. Ultimately, this approach saves you time in life, allowing you to do more of what you love, whether that activity happens to take place in or out of the kitchen.

Preparing meals may not come naturally to you—you might find the planning, shopping, and executing aspects of it quite stressful. You might be a home cook out of sheer necessity, not out of joy. In your endeavors to spend the shortest time in the kitchen, you might resolve to put together meals with conveniently precooked ingredients, such as canned beans and tomato sauce. One of the main critiques my readers offered about my first cookbook, *What to Eat for How You Feel*, was the time-consuming nature of the recipes, because I ask the

reader to make everything from scratch. I've been a vegetarian for more than thirty years, and I understand that washing and chopping vegetables is more involved than cooking a piece of meat. If you are new to Ayurvedic cooking and feel intimidated by its unfamiliar ingredients and cooking techniques, I encourage you to incorporate them incrementally. Don't start making tamarind paste from scratch. Instead, get comfortable with presoaking your beans and nuts. When that becomes second nature to you, implement another practice; for example, making your own almond milk.

Freshly prepared ingredients and meals are indispensable in a healthy diet. This is why, instead of opening a can of beans, I ask you to soak dried beans and cook them yourself. Instead of buying almond milk, I teach you how to make it at home. I encourage you to grind your spices instead of buying them powdered. Yes, it takes more time to cook from scratch, but you will get remarkable returns. Give yourself the opportunity and time to transition to this way of cooking. Your food will be at its highest nutritional, medicinal, and culinary value.

I observe this with my students all of the time—they are astonished by the empowerment they feel from learning to make staple recipes. Their excitement translates into commitment and consistency with their home cooking as well as motivation to teach others, including their children, how to enjoy and benefit from these recipes.

To cook healthy meals in less time, you must develop habits of efficiency, and these habits often require a specific sequence: first you plan, then you shop, then you cook, and while cooking, you clean. Believe it or not, you can find relaxation in this entire process when you approach it with curiosity and mindfulness. It all starts with planning. Just as you map out your route to get from your house to a new destination, doing a little preparation for your next meal will allow you to effortlessly make a quick, nutritious dish in minutes. It may take some trial and error to find the time-saving techniques that transform your cooking into an eloquent dance of creativity and exploration. For me, my dance is dictated by the flow of my week: on busy days at the restaurant and cooking school, I tend to utilize more of a "quick-cooking mode." On off days, I balance this with a "take-my-time cooking mode," when I revel in recipe development and experimentation and making additional treats. Here are some tips to inspire your dance:

PLAN: Become familiar with the recipes, decide on quantities, and acquire the ingredients and equipment you need for the week.

MAKE STAPLES: Once a month, make ghee and spice blends; every two to three days, make paneer cheese, yogurt, or nut milks—whichever you need for the week.

PREP:

- Soak your lentils or beans overnight, then rinse, drain, and cover them in the refrigerator until you're ready to cook them.

- Chop vegetables the day before using them, especially the vegetables that need peeling. (Chopping vegetables in smaller pieces will speed up their cooking time.)

- My friend Sasha Hynes shares this trick: If you are not able to grow your own herbs, consider sorting and washing store-bought herbs ahead of time, then storing them all together in a salad spinner in the refrigerator for several days.

- Prepare vegetables that appear in later steps while your first step of cooking is underway. For example, in the Spring Greens Soup recipe (page 108), you can wash, cut, and sauté the greens while the millet is boiling.

- Boil a pot or kettle of water, and use it to expedite your cooking of soups, grains, vegetables, or teas.

SELECT: When you only have fifteen minutes to fix a meal, choose quick-cooking vegetables that do not need peeling, such as zucchini or yellow squash, asparagus, fennel, cabbage, leafy greens, green beans, cauliflower, or broccoli.

CLEAN AS YOU GO: There is always a minute or two during cooking or before continuing on to the next step of the recipe to clean and organize the kitchen.

COOK IN A TIMELY SEQUENCE: Consider any required soaking time, and start with the dishes that take longer to cook (e.g., soups, stews, braises, roasts) and that need to cool down to be served at room temperature or chilled (e.g., desserts, chutneys). Then make the faster cooking dishes that are best served steamy hot (e.g., grains, vegetables). If you're cooking an elaborate dinner, make desserts, broths, sauces, or beverages earlier in the day or the day before.

USE A SLOW COOKER: Set up the slow cooker in the evening to either have breakfast ready upon rising or lunch ready to pack into a thermos that you can take with you for a hot meal later in the day.

USE A PRESSURE COOKER: When you simply need a meal cooked in a short amount of time, use a pressure cooker set to low pressure. Although pressure-cooked food is harder to digest, it is better than eating leftovers or unwholesome food.

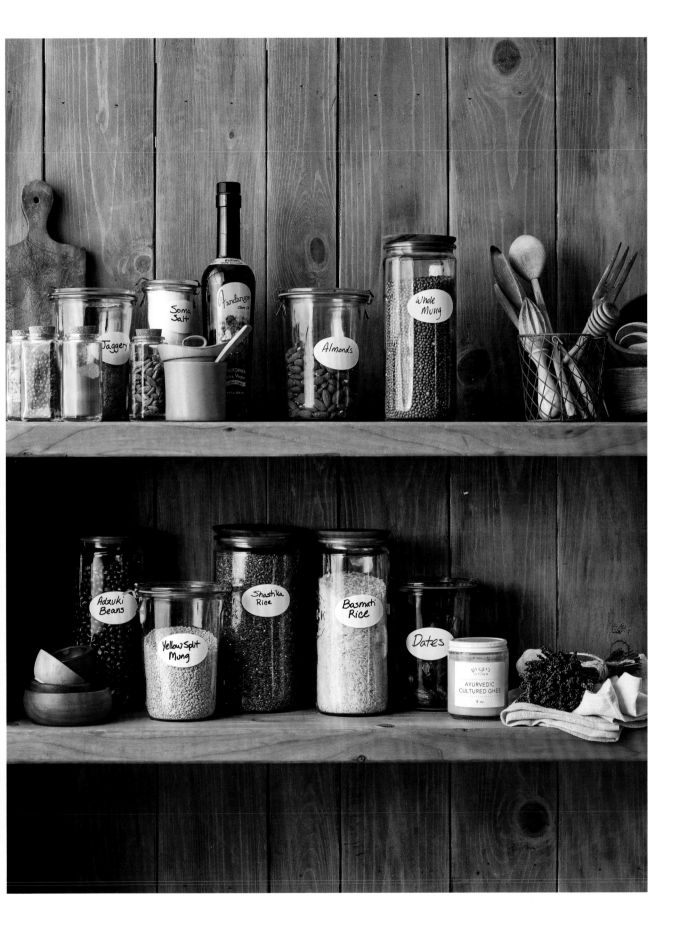

about the recipes and ingredient profiles

I want to help you deepen your relationship with individual foods by getting to know their attributes, healing benefits, and when to eat or not eat them. To do this, I organized the recipe section of this book by ingredient. In *What to Eat for How You Feel*, my recipes are organized according to season, a perspective that Ayurveda highly regards. Although seasonal eating is not the focus of this book, it remains an aspect worth considering. Therefore, at the top of each recipe, you will see the season(s) in which I recommend it is best to eat most often. I also share tips for cooking and digestibility and then give you one or more recipes starring the profiled ingredient.

There is so much to be said about each ingredient. Because modern nutrition facts are easily accessible and are often not Ayurveda's focus when learning about an ingredient, I chose to omit this information here and instead present the facts given in the classical Ayurvedic texts, such as *Charaka Samhita*, *Ashtanga Hridayam*, *Bhava Prakasha*, and the pharmacopeia compilation *Dravya-guna-vijnana*. Students of Ayurveda often look at the world through the attributes that an object or situation embodies. In the context of food, these attributes include taste, qualities, metabolic effect, post-digestive effect, and healing benefits. (I elaborate on them in *What to Eat for How You Feel*.) This less-familiar but valuable knowledge will help you understand how an ingredient interacts with your physiology, which will then make it easier for you to decide whether it is your balancing food.

The Ayurvedic classical texts describe ingredients that thrived in the lands of ancient India. Many of these ingredients are not available today, and for those that are, their attributes might be slightly different because of changes in their habitat, such as soil, climate, environmental pollution, and farming practices. Turmeric grown in South India will have a slightly different color, taste, metabolic effect, and nutrient value than turmeric grown in Hawaii or California. Still, the general attributes of turmeric being bitter and heating remain.

In addition to the currently unavailable or the different varieties of ingredients, today we are familiar with many wholesome foods that were never mentioned in these classical texts because they were not native to the Indian subcontinent. This does not mean that we cannot or should not incorporate them into our Ayurvedic meals. One of the main Ayurvedic principles of compatibility is to use locally grown foods. Olives, olive oil, and artichokes are wholesome and welcome on my Ayurveda table. So are quinoa, asparagus, celery root, kale, and so many more. Although not described by the ancient authors, they are still nutritious and health-promoting.

I've chosen to profile ingredients that are available to us today. I encourage you to read an ingredient's profile before you cook with it in a recipe for the first time. All of the recipes are lactovegetarian, and most are vegan friendly. I'm also proud to feature the accomplishments of some of our ANACT graduates by including a few of the recipes they created in the training.

following a recipe

Read the whole recipe before you start making it; within it, you'll discover the many details and tips you need to succeed. When you plan, make sure to note the soaking, prep, and cooking times. These times are approximate and vary according to several factors, such as the size of your pot and burner, the level of heat used, and the quantity of food you prepare. Follow your intuition as you adjust to these variables.

GF = gluten free

DF = dairy free

Follow the dosha balancing variations based on the dosha you feel is high for you right now and wish to lower. For example, if you are making the Millet Pilaf with Grated Carrots (page 60) and feel that your Vata is in excess, it would be best for you to adapt the recipe with my "Vata Balancing" suggestion listed under the ingredient list. In this case, you would add nuts to the recipe, which help reduce or pacify the Vata dosha.

It is very important that you enjoy the taste and the looks of your food. Use my recipes as guidelines and feel free to adjust the tastes and seasonings of the dish to your liking. If you prefer it a little more sour, add more lime juice. If it tastes bland, add a little more salt. If you prefer your dish extra spicy, add more chile or ginger. Ayurveda highlights "palatability" as one important food compatibility criteria—taking pleasure in your food will make it more digestible. As for applying all other compatibility principles to each recipe (see Ayurvedic Food Compatibility Chart, page 244), do not worry—I've taken care of that for you.

Now, what ingredients do you feel like cooking with today?

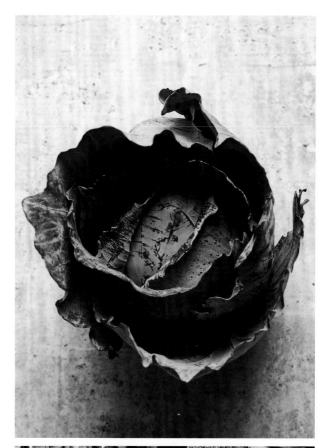

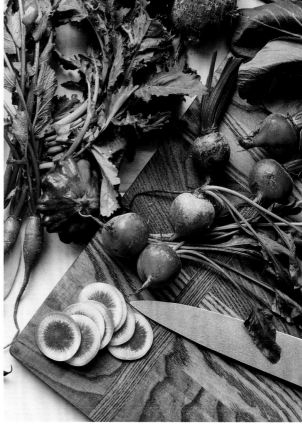

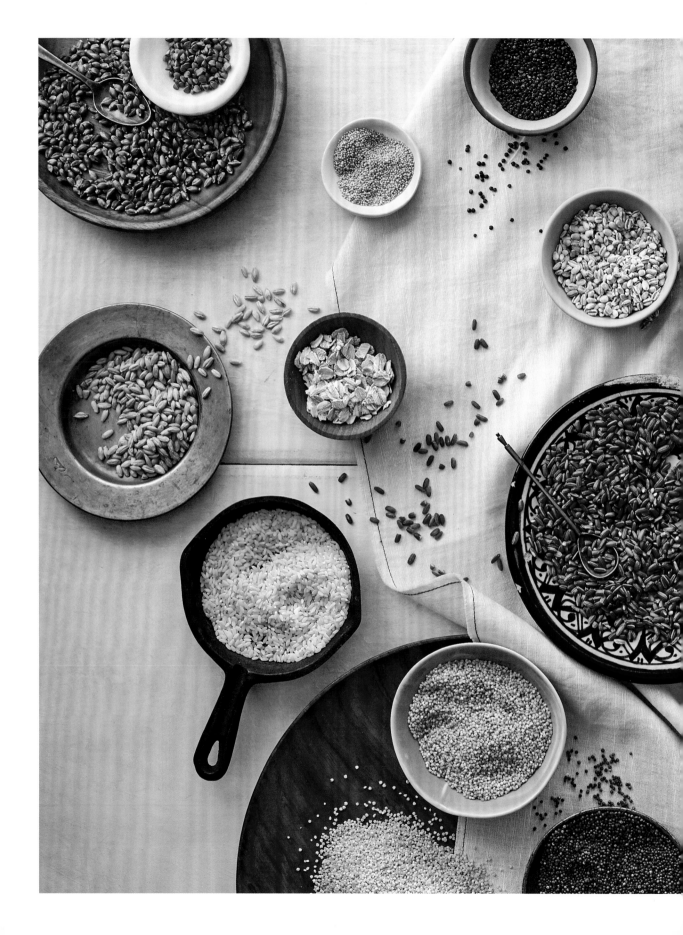

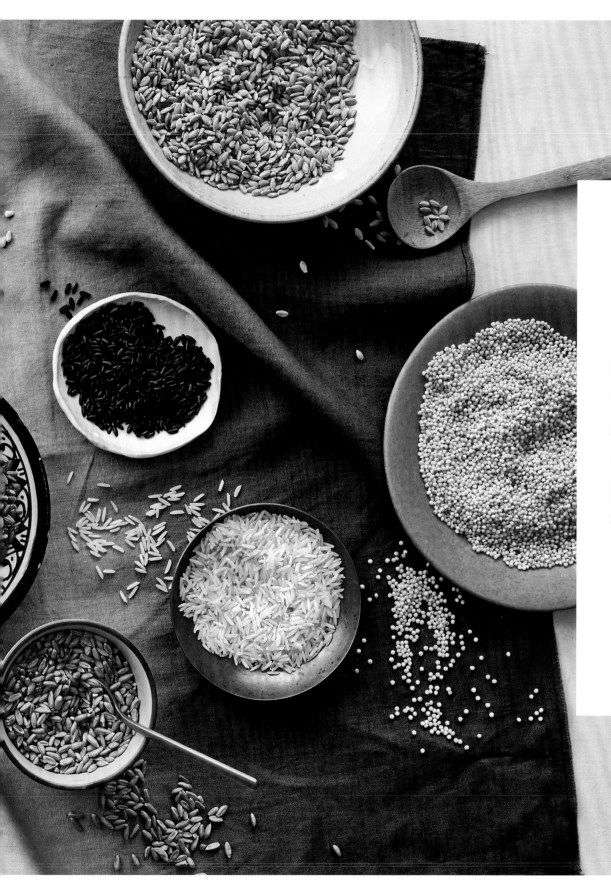

GRAINS

I think of grains as the baseline for human nutrition. They have been the primary source for building and strengthening our bodies since the beginning of evolution. It's no wonder, because whole grains contain all essential nutrients for our sustenance: complex carbohydrates, fiber, protein, minerals, vitamins, and fats.

Despite some modern opinions, Ayurveda stands by the concept that we all need to eat grains to efficiently give our bodies those nutrients; we just need to determine which ones are the most suitable for us, and Ayurvedic guidelines can help us do that. In my case, I need a grain with every meal to keep my Vata grounded and my Pitta satiated; I'd feel weak if I didn't have a grain. If you're of a Kapha constitution, you likely need less grains and could omit them from your meal on the days you feel sluggish. As you study the attributes of the grains I outline in this section, you will be able to select the grains that are most suitable for you right now.

Ayurveda calls grains *shuka-dhanya*, or members of the sharp-grass family (exceptions are amaranth, buckwheat, and quinoa). In the Ayurvedic texts there are detailed descriptions of groups of grains, their attributes, and their daily or medicinal uses. The authors of the classical texts always considered the properties of unadulterated whole grains. The practice

of refining and genetically altering grains started in the mid-twentieth century, when large corporations opted to produce food for profit, not for health and nutrition. Soon after that, people began developing all kinds of chronic gut and blood sugar disorders that continue to trouble us today.

Refined (and often artificially enriched) flour is the form of grains that have been denatured the most. While refining extends the shelf life and makes pastries attractive and enjoyable, the *ama* accumulated from regularly eating white flour can cause systemic digestive issues and food allergies. If you're on a quest to improve your health, it will serve you well to say goodbye to the bread, pizza, pasta, cakes, cookies, and other similar foods made from refined flour. Go back to whole grains and feel whole again.

You could seek out these whole grain baked foods from holistic grocers and healthy restaurants, but the quality and healing benefits will no doubt be greater when you make them yourself. Since you're reading this book, I imagine you like to cook. So to take your healthy baking a nudge further, I'd suggest investing in a grain mill to make fresh flour and cracked grains (cut oats, for example). Flour starts to spoil within a couple of days of milling it, which is why most flours on the market have preservatives in them. Baking with fresh-milled flour not only lends a superb flavor, texture, and nutrition to your pastries—it also requires less storage space. In my home pantry and at Divya's Kitchen, I keep airtight containers with the whole grains of einkorn, spelt, rye, barley, millet, oats, sorghum, and a few others. Whenever I need flour, I grind grain berries for only as much flour as the recipe calls for. I also have a grain flaker to make fresh rolled oats and barley or quinoa flakes whenever I need them. In this way, I don't have to worry about having separate containers for flour, flakes, and their whole grain version or about the extra refrigerated storage space for my flours. Whole grains have a very

long shelf life, and they are also cheaper than flour. See Sources (page 248) for my favorite stone-grinding grain mill.

general tips for digesting grains

- Buy organic and free from chemical or genetic intervention.

- Soak in advance. The amount of time depends on the grain.

- Cook them to increase the bioavailability of their nutrients.

- Eat them freshly cooked, as leftover reheated grains cause a lot of *ama*.

- Chew them well to produce their digestive enzyme ptyalin (made only in the mouth).

- Eat only one type per meal, especially if your digestion is weak.

- If your digestion is very weak, avoid flour because it is harder to digest than the full grain.

BARLEY

Barley is one of the oldest grains on earth, originating in Southwest Asia more than eighty-five hundred years ago. Ayurvedic doctors have been using it in dietary and clinical protocols for centuries. Today it is mostly cooked in soups or malted into syrup, beer, or whiskey. I regularly include barley flakes in my breakfast meals, whole barley in my soups, and barley flour in my baking.

BOTANICAL NAME ● *Hordeum vulgare*

SANSKRIT NAME ● *Yava*

AYURVEDIC ATTRIBUTES

TASTE ● lightly astringent, sweet

QUALITIES ● dry, rough, heavy to digest

METABOLIC EFFECT ● cooling

POST-DIGESTIVE EFFECT ● pungent or sweet

DOSHA EFFECTS ● alleviates Kapha and Pitta disorders, increases Vata in the colon

HEALING BENEFITS ● promotes stability and stamina for both the body and mind, acts as a diuretic, enhances complexion, alleviates ulcers, stimulates the appetite, binds toxins in the colon and blood, regulates blood sugar, lowers cholesterol, can have a constipating effect (when eaten cooked), works as prebiotic, is an aphrodisiac

WHOLE (HULLED) BARLEY ● It has a light brownish color. The grain's outer husk is removed but the bran remains intact—this is the most nutritious form of barley (13% protein). It cooks in about 60 minutes and is quite chewy and more medicinal than pearled barley.

PEARLED BARLEY ● It is whitish in color because its bran has been polished off. It cooks in about 35 minutes, and it is easier to digest, making it useful for people with slow digestion.

BARLEY FLAKES ● These are rolled from whole barley groats, with their nutrition intact. They cook in only 10 minutes and make an excellent breakfast cereal, granola, grain dish, or soup thickener.

SOURCING

● Look for any of the above barley options in your local health food store, farmers market, or online. It is important to buy organic barley because the nonorganic options are loaded with harmful chemicals.

SEASON

● Barley is most balancing to our mind and body in cold temperatures, but it's also fine to occasionally eat in the summer.

DIGESTIBILITY

● Barley has small amounts of gluten, and I've met many gluten-sensitive people who do not react to organic barley. To better digest this ancient grain (especially for Vata types), always cook it with spices, such as kalonji, fennel, coriander, curry leaves, ginger, chiles, or cumin. For using barley in a sweet dish, add cinnamon, cardamom, or cloves.

COOKING TIPS

Whether you're using whole or pearled barley, always soak it for at least 8 hours or overnight. This will not only reduce cooking time but will also enhance digestibility.

EAT BARLEY WHENEVER YOU NEED TO

● release water retention,

● soothe a sore throat,

● strengthen your voice,

● stop a runny nose,

● reduce lung congestion,

● relieve cough, and/or

● build strength.

COOK BARLEY WATER WHENEVER YOU NEED TO

● soothe the mind and build strength after surgery, prolonged illness, or food poisoning,

● flush out kidney stones,

● reduce a urinary tract infection,

● reduce gut inflammation,

● convalesce after serious illness or surgery.

minestrone

SERVES 5 to 6 ● SOAK: 8 hours or overnight ● PREP: 20 minutes ● COOK: about 1 hour ● DF ●
FALL-WINTER-SPRING

I must confess: my fondness for Italian-style cooking has secretly grown into a romantic relationship. Minestrone literally translates to "big soup." With a legume, grain, and vegetables all in one pot, minestrone to me is the Italian version of Indian kitchari. In this recipe, I add a couple of Indian spices to influence a digestion-supporting relationship and facilitate the connection of two cuisines to develop into a marriage of flavors. And similar to kitchari, minestrone can be considered a complete meal. The beauty of the recipe is that you can adjust the texture to your liking and the vegetables to the season. The traditional consistency is pretty thick, but it can vary from creamy to brothy depending on your choice of ingredients.

Enjoy this nourishing soup with Basil-Parsley Pesto (page 217), Vegan and Gluten-Free Paratha Flatbread (page 56), or Steamed Kale Salad (page 109).

½ cup chickpeas, adzuki beans, or green lentils, soaked in water for at least 8 hours or overnight, rinsed, and drained

2¼ teaspoons salt, divided

2 tablespoons olive oil or ghee

1 tablespoon thinly slivered fresh ginger

1 small green Indian or Thai chile, seeded and minced

½ teaspoon ground cumin

Tiny pinch of asafoetida

¼ cup whole barley, soaked in water at least 8 hours or overnight, rinsed, and drained

1 cup peeled and chopped (½-inch pieces) taro root or turnip

1 cup thinly sliced green cabbage

1 cup peeled and diced (¼-inch) carrots (1 medium carrot)

½ cup sliced celery

2 tablespoons pulp from fresh sweet Thai tamarind pods (optional; do not use store-bought tamarind paste)

1 tablespoon dried basil

1 teaspoon dried oregano

1 cup diced (¼-inch) zucchini (1 medium zucchini)

GARNISHES

2 tablespoons chopped fresh basil leaves

2 tablespoons chopped fresh parsley leaves

2 teaspoons fresh lime juice, or to taste

¼ teaspoon freshly ground black pepper

Olive oil or melted ghee

FOR VATA BALANCING: Green lentils would be easiest for you to digest.

FOR PITTA BALANCING: Omit the green chile.

FOR KAPHA BALANCING: Increase the green chile, if you like.

CONTINUED

1. In a 2-quart saucepan, cover the beans or lentils with 2 inches water and bring to a boil. Lower the heat, partially cover, and simmer for 30 to 45 minutes (depending on the bean or lentil you're using). Add 1 teaspoon of the salt and continue to cook for another 10 to 15 minutes, until the beans are soft and start to open up. (You can also slow cook them for about 4 hours.) Remove from the heat and set them aside in their cooking water until they are ready to go into the soup.

2. Meanwhile, in a 4-quart saucepan, heat the olive oil over low heat. Add the ginger, chile, cumin, and asafoetida, then the barley, taro, cabbage, carrots, and celery and sauté for 5 minutes. Add the sweet tamarind pulp, dried basil and oregano, the remaining 1¼ teaspoons salt, and 4 cups water. Bring to a boil, then lower the heat to low, cover, and simmer for about 20 minutes, until the vegetables are tender. Add the zucchini and cooked beans (with their cooking water) and continue to simmer for another 10 minutes, or until all the ingredients are tender and the texture is medium thick—a comforting creamy feel. If you prefer yours more brothy, adjust the consistency and taste by adding hot water and more salt.

3. Garnish each bowl with fresh basil and parsley, a sprinkle of lime juice, a few turns of the peppermill, and a drizzle of olive oil. Serve hot.

VARIATIONS

For a gluten-free option, substitute 2 tablespoons rinsed white quinoa for the barley. Add it with the vegetables in Step 2.

For other vegetable options, try using daikon radish, celery root, or kohlrabi, to name a few.

For a beautiful orange-pink color, substitute ¼ cup peeled and diced red beets for ¼ cup of the carrots.

How to Make Barley Water

Cook ¼ cup whole barley in 4 cups water for 30 minutes. Strain, cool down to warm, and add a pinch of freshly ground black pepper and a splash of fresh lime juice. Sip slowly between meals or when you're recovering from an illness or surgery and need to have a light meal or a meal substitute.

Opposite: Minestrone, Vegan and Gluten-Free Bread, Basil-Parsley Pesto

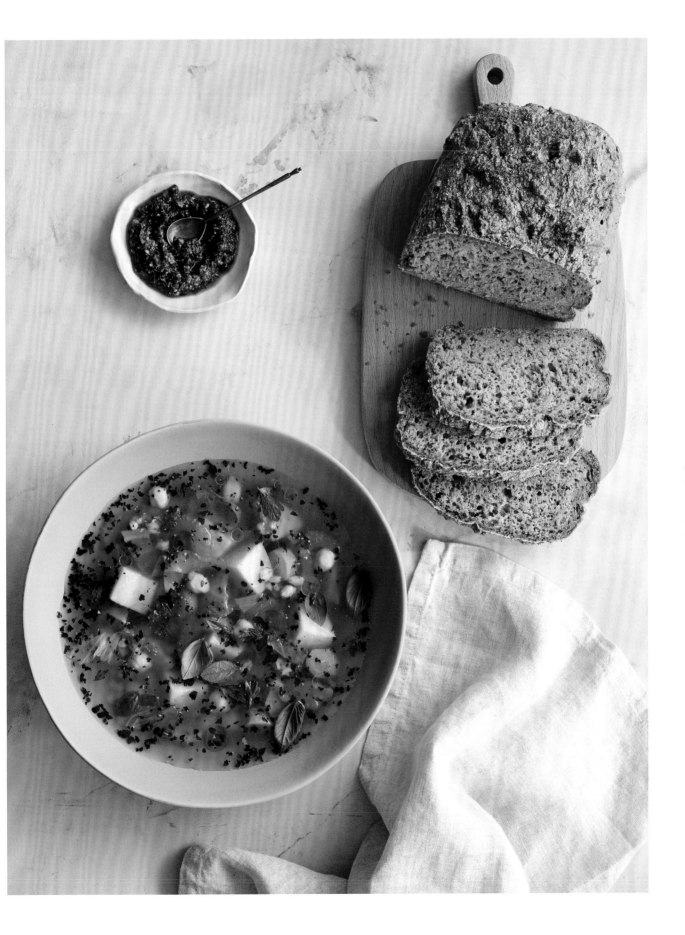

care for oily skin

"If you won't put it in your mouth, don't put it on your skin." This was one of the first guidelines I learned about Ayurvedic skin care. The principle is that our skin absorbs substances that land on it, be they nutrients or pollutants. Chemical skin care products may offer quick, short-term improvement, but once they are applied to the skin, they enter the blood stream, slowly contributing to a buildup of toxicity in the body. That is not the case with skin products made from all-natural ingredients, such as flours, herbs, and essential oils.

You can create cleansers, moisturizers, masks, and creams right in your kitchen! With the recipes below (inspired by Pratima Raichur's classic book *Absolute Beauty*), you can use barley in a daily skin care routine to target oily skin. For best results, make yours with organic ingredients.

You'll find cleanser recipes for sensitive skin on page 93 and for dry skin on page 192.

skin cleansing powder for oily skin

This powder offers a gentle exfoliation and a deep wash of the top layer of the facial skin. Use it daily in the morning and evening.

4 teaspoons almond meal

1 tablespoon barley flour

2 teaspoons chickpea or lentil flour

1 teaspoon dried lemon peel powder (see Note)

TO MAKE: Using a mortar and pestle, mix all the ingredients. Store in a dry, airtight container away from light (I keep mine in the bathroom vanity).

TO USE: Scoop ½ teaspoon of the cleansing powder onto your palm and add enough warm water to make a thin but not runny paste. Apply the paste all over your face and gently massage it in for about 1 minute. Do not scrub. Rinse well with warm (not hot) water. Let your skin air dry. Follow up with a toner and moisturizer of your choice.

NOTE: If you can't source dried lemon peel powder, make it yourself: Dry the chopped peel of 2 organic lemons in a dehydrator at 95°F for about 24 hours or on a baking sheet in the oven at 200°F for about 2 hours, until it dries completely. Grind to a powder and store in an airtight container.

probiotic mask for oily skin

This mask offers deep cleaning of the pores and restores the friendly bacteria on your facial skin. Use it once or twice a week.

1 teaspoon Skin Cleansing Powder for Oily Skin (see recipe to the left)

Plain yogurt (enough to create a medium-thick paste)

TO MAKE: In a small bowl, mix the Skin Cleansing Powder for Oily Skin with enough yogurt to create a medium-thick paste.

TO USE: Apply the mask on your face, leave it for 10 minutes, then rinse off with warm water. Let your skin air dry. Follow up with a toner and moisturizer of your choice.

BUCKWHEAT

Although not mentioned in the classical Sanskrit texts (probably because it did not grow in India back in the day), buckwheat is an important grain (technically a seed) to highlight today, as it is widely used in gluten-free recipes. Buckwheat is highly nutritious and supports our health in many ways. Give it a try and see how it works for you.

BOTANICAL NAME ● *Fagopyrum esculentum*

SANSKRIT NAME ● Unknown

AYURVEDIC ATTRIBUTES

TASTE ● astringent, sweet, pungent

QUALITIES ● heavy, drying

METABOLIC EFFECT ● heating

POST-DIGESTIVE EFFECT ● sweet

DOSHA EFFECTS ● increases Vata and Pitta, reduces Kapha

HEALING BENEFITS ● supports the large intestine, has a long transition through the gut and is therefore low glycemic, acts as a blood builder, dilates blood vessels, improves circulation

COMMON FORMS OF BUCKWHEAT

RAW BUCKWHEAT GROATS ● They are of tan-greenish color and mild flavor. I usually use them to make fresh buckwheat flour or I dry roast them before cooking them as a grain dish.

ROASTED BUCKWHEAT GROATS ● Also known as *kasha*, these are roasted groats of a rich brown color and stronger, nutty flavor. My favorite kasha is the Russian type, which is dark brown and cooks perfectly into a fluffy grain dish without getting mushy.

CREAM OF BUCKWHEAT OR BUCKWHEAT GRITS ● These forms are a coarse cut of the groats, usually cooked into a breakfast cereal.

BUCKWHEAT FLOUR ● The flour is made from raw groats. Its color varies from light to dark depending on how much of its black hull was ground into the flour. A dish baked with dark buckwheat flour will have a dark chocolate-like color.

SEASON

● Because of buckwheat's drying and heating attributes, the best season to enjoy it is spring, when we experience increased Kapha qualities in our body.

DIGESTIBILITY

● Buckwheat is heavy to digest, so it is better to avoid when you have a low appetite.

● To make it easier on your stomach, always cook it with ghee or olive oil to balance its drying effect; add dried herbs such as thyme, savory, basil, or marjoram; garnish it with fresh dill or cilantro; add spices such as coriander, fennel, fresh ginger, or cinnamon stick.

COOKING TIPS

● Dry roast raw buckwheat groats by adding them to a skillet and shaking them over medium-high heat until the groats turn brown and aromatic.

● I use a 1:3 ratio of well-roasted buckwheat groats to boiling hot water when cooking them as a grain dish.

● Use it as a substitute for rice or quinoa in pilafs, salads, and stuffing.

● Buckwheat flour binds well, making it a good gluten-free substitute for wheat in pastries or flatbreads.

EAT BUCKWHEAT WHEN YOU NEED TO

● balance oily skin,

● keep your blood sugar in check,

● mitigate varicose veins,

● improve circulation,

● lower your cholesterol or blood pressure,

● counteract damage from radiation,

● improve your blood count,

● build your stamina, and/or

● strengthen your bones.

gluten-free paratha flatbread

MAKES 8 flatbreads • PREP: 20 minutes • COOK: about 35 minutes • GF, DF • YEAR-ROUND •
Photograph on page 129

This recipe is by Bijal Nishit Shukla (@HealthyBraja), a graduate of our Ayurvedic Nutrition and Culinary Training and dear friend of mine. She has mastered every possible Indian flatbread and created this gluten-free recipe for her son, who developed a wheat allergy at an early age.

If you dread making flatbreads because they seem messy and time-consuming, you're right. But partially right. In time, you will be able to effortlessly roll them into perfectly round disks and have fun cooking them. It just takes practice.

Flatbreads are the best type of bread because they are easy to digest and free from leaveners. I find it most enjoyable to smell the aroma of a piping hot, soft layered paratha, break a piece of it with my fingers, and dip it into a sauce or cooked vegetables—a simple luxury displayed in every Indian household.

Serve Gluten-Free Paratha Flatbread with any meal. You can also use them as shells for tacos or tostadas.

¾ cup (118 grams) buckwheat flour, plus
    ¼ cup for dusting

1 cup (113 grams) amaranth or millet flour

1 tablespoon minced fresh mint or cilantro
    leaves

1 teaspoon salt

2 tablespoons olive oil

1 tablespoon ghee or coconut oil

1. In a medium bowl, mix the 1 cup buckwheat flour, amaranth flour, mint, and salt. Rub in the olive oil, then add about ⅔ cup room temperature water (or as much as needed, depending on the flour), kneading the ingredients into a smooth and soft dough that is pliable but not sticky, about 5 minutes.

2. Divide the dough into 8 equal portions and roll each one into a ball. Cover the balls with a damp kitchen towel.

3. Dust a smooth surface with the ¼ cup buckwheat flour and, using a small rolling pin, roll each ball into a 6-inch or so disk (about 2 millimeters thick). If your disks are cracking on the edges, your dough needs a little more water.

4. Line a tortilla warmer, a basket, or a wide enough saucepan with a clean tea towel for storing the cooked flatbreads.

5. To cook the parathas: Preheat a cast-iron griddle over medium heat and brush it with a little ghee. Place one paratha in the middle of the griddle and lower the heat to medium-low. Once the top side begins to bubble, brush it with a little ghee, then flip it with a spatula. Cook the second side for another minute or two, until it has reddish-brown spots. Brush the top and edges of the bread with a little ghee, then gently flip the paratha back to the first side. Cook for a few more seconds. Your paratha may puff up partially—that's a good sign. Slip the cooked paratha into the prepared tortilla warmer or basket and fold the towel to cover the bread. On to cooking the next paratha.

6. Keep the parathas stacked and hot and serve them immediately.

vegan and gluten-free bread

MAKES 1 loaf of bread ● **SOAK:** 30 minutes ● **PREP:** 20 minutes ● **BAKE:** 60 minutes ● **GF, DF** ●
YEAR-ROUND ● Photograph on page 53

This is a variation of a recipe by Michaela Vais from her ElaVegan blog. I've always admired her creativity and her remarkable productivity in publishing recipes. I was excited about this recipe because I was looking for a delicious vegan and gluten-free bread to serve at Divya's Kitchen. I think it is a rare achievement to make such bread very spongy and "toastable" without any yeast. On our restaurant menu, we serve it as Gluten-Free Toast.

This bread is of brownish color, moist, soft, and springy, yet it holds well when sliced (thank you, psyllium husk powder!). I prefer toasting the slices on a cast-iron griddle with ghee or coconut oil. If you try that, you'll notice that the slices are very "thirsty" for oil. Many friends tell me that this bread reminds them of a Jewish rye bread. It is very fragrant, chewy, and filling.

Enjoy Vegan and Gluten-Free Bread with any soup or stew, or use it as a base for sandwiches and more.

3 tablespoons (30 grams) psyllium husk powder

1 cup (100 grams) besan or garbanzo flour

⅔ cup (100 grams) white rice flour, plus more for dusting

½ cup (50 grams) oat flour

⅓ cup (50 grams) buckwheat flour

⅓ cup (40 grams) tapioca starch, plus more as needed

1 tablespoon caraway seeds

1⅛ teaspoons salt

1 teaspoon baking powder

¼ teaspoon baking soda

Olive oil

1½ tablespoons apple cider vinegar

1. In a medium bowl, combine 2 cups room temperature water with the psyllium husk powder and whisk thoroughly. Set aside for 30 minutes, or until the liquid thickens and turns gel-like.

2. Meanwhile, in another medium bowl, mix the besan flour, rice flour, oat flour, buckwheat flour, tapioca starch, caraway seeds, salt, baking powder, and baking soda.

3. Preheat the oven to 350°F. Grease a 1½-quart bread pan with olive oil and dust with rice flour.

4. Whisk the vinegar into the psyllium gel mix, then fold the wet mixture into the dry to form a dough. Knead the dough with your hands for 5 to 10 minutes, until it comes together and is soft, pliable, and sticky but still easy to shape. Alternatively, make the dough in a standing mixer. If the dough is too wet and sticky, knead in 1 to 2 tablespoons tapioca starch. If it is too dry (not sticky at all), add a little water. Wet your fingers and shape the dough into the prepared pan. Bake for 60 minutes, or until a toothpick or skewer inserted in the middle of the bread comes out clean.

5. Let the bread cool in the pan for 10 minutes, then transfer to a cooling rack. Let it cool down completely before slicing. Please keep in mind that this bread is moist, so if you slice it while it's still warm, it will look pasty.

6. To store: Wrap the bread tightly in plastic wrap and keep it at room temperature for up to three days.

MILLET

Don't be too quick to reject millet from your pantry and label it birdseed! You might be surprised at how much this ancient grain can do for you. Among cereal grains, millet is very rich in iron, calcium, amino acids, and protein. Unlike rice, which requires a lot of water, attention, and cultivation techniques to properly grow, millet is in the group of grasses that does not require a lot of water to grow, making it easy to cultivate in hot or cold regions with less rainfall.

BOTANICAL NAME ● *Poaceae*

SANSKRIT NAME FOR THE GROUP OF MILLETS ● *trina-dhanya* ("a tiny seed that brings wealth to your body")

AYURVEDIC ATTRIBUTES

TASTE ● sweet, astringent

QUALITIES ● light (in weight), heavy to digest

METABOLIC EFFECT ● cooling (some varieties are heating)

POST-DIGESTIVE EFFECT ● sweet (pungent in some varieties)

DOSHA EFFECTS ● increases Vata, reduces Kapha and Pitta

HEALING BENEFITS ● has a scraping effect on the intestinal mucus lining, withholds nutrients, acts as a diuretic, causes dryness in the body, acts as a decongestant, cleanses the blood, regulates blood sugar, lowers cholesterol

COMMON FORMS OF MILLET

PEARL MILLET

BOTANICAL NAME ● *Cenchrus americanus* or *Pennisetum glaucum*

SANSKRIT NAME ● *Ikshupattra*

This is perhaps the most commonly used millet in the world. It varies in color, with pale yellow being the most popular. It has a cooling metabolic effect.

FOXTAIL MILLET

BOTANICAL NAME ● *Setaria italica*

SANSKRIT NAME ● *Kangu, Priyangu*

This is the second-most widely used type of millet in the world, grown primarily in eastern Asia. In the US, it is grown in Colorado, Nebraska, and the Dakotas. It comes in black, red, white, or yellow colors; Ayurveda considers yellow to be the best.

The classical Ayurveda texts describe foxtail millet as heating and heavier to digest than other millet varieties. It gives body strength, greatly reduces Kapha, and a topical application of its paste (see recipe below) can help speed up the healing of fractured bones.

PROSO MILLET

BOTANICAL NAME ● *Panicum miliaceum*

SANSKRIT NAME ● *Chinaka*

This is the most commonly used millet in the US. Its seeds are small, round, and yellow in color. It is slightly heating, and its properties are similar to foxtail millet.

KODO MILLET

BOTANICAL NAME ● *Paspalum scrobiculatum*

SANSKRIT NAME ● *Kodrava*

This hardy grain grows primarily in Nepal and Africa. With its light, drying, and cooling properties, it balances Pitta and Kapha and is quite aggravating for Vata.

BARNYARD MILLET

BOTANICAL NAME ● *Echinochloa*

SANSKRIT NAME ● *Shyamaka*

Rich in calcium, iron, and fiber, this millet variety is often used as a replacement for rice and on the special fasting days known as Ekadashi. It is beneficial in managing diabetes and in reducing weight and symptoms of rheumatoid arthritis. Because of its highly absorbent nature, barnyard millet is also used to absorb and eliminate poisons from the body.

FINGER MILLET

BOTANICAL NAME ● *Eleusine coracana*

SANSKRIT NAME ● *Ragi*

There is no surprise that this red colored millet is widely grown in India and cooked as a daily staple in parts of South India. Being low glycemic and high in fiber, finger millet is excellent for diabetic and high cholesterol conditions. It is rich in calcium, iron, protein, and other nutrients, and this is why it is used to increase hemoglobin in blood, strengthen bones, or heal bone fractures. It has a cooling metabolic effect, balances Pitta and Kapha, and is best tolerated by high Vata.

SOURCING

● There are different types of millet grown all over the world, so look for the varieties that are local to your area. In the US, proso millet is what you will commonly find in health food stores. The other varieties of millet mentioned above are available in Indian grocery stores and online (see Sources, page 248).

● Shelf life varies depending on the type of millet and its fat content—the higher the percentage of fat, the longer it stores. I buy the less enduring millets in small quantity and keep them refrigerated in airtight containers. Discard millet grains or flour that have turned rancid or bitter.

SEASON

● Millet is most balancing in spring or during humid periods.

DIGESTIBILITY

Compared to rice, millet is heavier to digest because it has higher amounts of protein and fat; because it is rich in fiber, it stays longer in the gut. To digest millet well, cook it with pungent spices such as chiles, ginger, green cardamom pods, cinnamon stick, and fenugreek.

COOKING TIPS

● Dry-toast the grains before adding water for a richer, nuttier flavor and fluffier texture.

● Use vegetable stock instead of water for cooking—this will enhance the otherwise neutral flavor of millet.

● Use a millet to water ratio of 1:2½ for a dry, fluffy texture and 1:3 for a creamy consistency.

● Use millet flour for cereal, flatbreads, pancakes, pastries, and more.

EAT MILLET WHEN YOU NEED TO

● clear congestion anywhere in the body,

● detox,

● lose weight,

● eat a sugar-balancing grain,

● clear *Candida albicans* overgrowth on your tongue and throat (thrush), and/or

● make a creamy cereal breakfast, especially in the spring.

CAUTION ● Do not overdo it, as excessive millet consumption can lead to depletion of the intestinal mucosal lining.

HOW TO MAKE MILLET WATER

Bring 3 cups water to a boil, add ½ cup finger millet, and simmer uncovered for 25 minutes. Drain into a vessel and add salt or honey for taste (optional).

DRINK MILLET WATER WHEN YOU WANT TO

● stop diarrhea,

● reduce heavy menstrual flow,

● stop runny eyes and nose,

● dry up nasal drip in the throat, and/or

● take in nourishment but cannot eat solid food.

HOW TO MAKE MILLET PASTE
(FOR CLOSED-FRACTURED BONES)

Mix foxtail millet flour and cold water to create a medium-thick paste. Spread it on some gauze, and gently wrap it around the fractured bone. Keep it on for 3 hours, discard the used paste, and gently wipe the affected area; repeat once a day for one to three weeks, or as needed.

millet pilaf with grated carrots

SERVES 1 to 2 ● PREP: 5 minutes ● COOK: 35 minutes ● GF, DF ● SPRING ● Photograph on page 64

I hope this recipe will help you fall in love with millet, especially foxtail millet, the way I did. I've had a few failed attempts to make millet exciting and palatable, but even after I learned how to cook it properly, I avoided millet because it makes my skin very dry. However, here you will experience millet to be quite Vata balancing and palatable. I must give credit to my mentor, the late Yamuna Devi, whose recipe is the inspiration behind the ingredient combination you'll find here. The spices help digest the grain's heaviness, and the fat, sesame seeds, and carrots add moisture and texture. The orange carrot shreds intertwine with the light yellow grains and the touches of dark brown raisins—this dish looks like a designer's piece of marble. Marbelous millet!

Millet Pilaf with Grated Carrots goes well with Green Tahini Sauce (page 219), Steamed Kale Salad (page 109), Dill-Mung Soup with Vegetable Noodles (page 89), or Sautéed Bitter Melon (page 135).

½ cup foxtail or proso millet
  (dry—do not rinse)

1 tablespoon ghee or olive oil

2 tablespoons white sesame seeds

3 whole cloves

3 black peppercorns

3 green cardamom pods, slightly crushed
  open on one end

1-inch piece cinnamon stick

¾ cup grated carrots

2 tablespoons Thompson raisins or currants

¾ teaspoon salt

1 tablespoon fresh orange juice

GARNISH

2 tablespoons whole cilantro leaves

FOR VATA OR PITTA BALANCING: Add 2 table-spoons slivered almonds or pine nuts with the spices in Step 3.

FOR KAPHA BALANCING: Enjoy as is or add a small seeded and minced green Indian or Thai chile with the spices in Step 3.

1. Dry-toast the millet in a small skillet over medium-low heat for 4 to 5 minutes, until the millet releases its aroma and it turns just a shade darker.

2. While you're toasting the millet, bring 1½ cups water to a boil.

3. In a medium sauté pan, heat the ghee over medium-low heat. Add the sesame seeds, cloves, peppercorns, cardamom pods, and cinnamon stick, and toast until the spices release their aroma, about 1 minute. Stir in the carrots, raisins, salt, toasted millet, and boiling water. Cover, lower the heat to low, and simmer for 20 minutes, or until the liquid has been absorbed and the grains are soft and fluffy. If some of the grains are still hard, add ¼ cup more hot water and continue to simmer for 5 minutes. The cooked millet will look like couscous—tiny grains, dry and fluffy.

4. Turn off the heat and let the grains rest for 5 minutes. Remove the whole spices from the surface of the millet, add the orange juice, and fluff with a fork.

5. Garnish with the cilantro. Serve hot.

RICE

The classical texts of Ayurveda describe the types of rice that were cultivated hundreds and thousands of years ago. Variations of some of the ancient rice grains can be found today, and some varieties are no longer available. Rice is the type of ingredient that has been frequently hybridized and genetically modified to serve high-yield manufacturing purposes. Agronomy modifications to rice continue to date, to achieve specific goals in regard to cultivation, yield, percentage of starch, length of growing, recipe usage, and more. Unfortunately, most of these altered types of rice do not fit within the rice properties described in the classical Ayurvedic texts.

In this section, I will briefly describe a few of the available rice varieties (or their modern cousins) mentioned in the classical Ayurvedic texts.

BOTANICAL NAME ● *Oryza sativa*

SANSKRIT NAME ● *Shali*

AYURVEDIC ATTRIBUTES

TASTE ● mildly sweet, with mildly astringent secondary taste (especially for red rice)

QUALITIES ● unctuous, soft, light to digest

METABOLIC EFFECT ● cooling

POST-DIGESTIVE EFFECT ● sweet

DOSHA EFFECTS ● balances Vata, Pitta, Kapha (high-starch varieties aggravate Kapha)

HEALING BENEFITS ● gives strength, nourishes the body, acts as an aphrodisiac, can have a constipating effect, acts as a diuretic

RED RICE

BOTANICAL NAME ● *Oryza punctata*

SANSKRIT NAME ● *Rakta-shali*

Considered the best rice of all, medium-grain red rice is made of a very balanced combination of the five material elements. It balances Vata, Pitta, and Kapha, relieves excessive thirst, and is suitable for daily consumption. It is good for the eyes and the voice.

Red Bhutanese rice comes close to the original variety described in the classical texts.

SHASHTIKA RICE

BOTANICAL NAME ● *Oryza sativa*

SANSKRIT NAME ● *Navara, Njvara*

Shashti in Sanskrit means "sixty." Unlike most rice grains that take one hundred to three hundred days to cultivate, shashtika rice is ready to harvest sixty days from planting. It is of reddish color, and it is used in a lot of medicinal recipes during Ayurvedic therapies, especially in South India.

Shashtika has similar properties to red rice, but it stays longer in the digestive tract; that's why it has lower glycemic index and is suitable for diabetic conditions.

WHITE BASMATI RICE

BOTANICAL NAME ● *Oryza sativa*

SANSKRIT NAME ● Unknown

This is a long-grain rice and easy to digest, but because of its higher starch content and its longer transition in the gut, some people might find it too heavy. Today's basmati rice is perhaps the closest cousin of the the Vrihi rice described in the classical texts: a rice harvested in the rainy season that yields white grains after pounding it (white without polishing it).

The best quality of basmati rice comes from North India and Pakistan. Favor organic basmati rice because many of the conventional varieties are genetically modified.

CONTINUED

BABY BASMATI RICE

BOTANICAL NAME ● *Oryza sativa*

BENGALI NAME ● *Kali Jeera*

This is a modern variety of a very small grain rice (almost the size of a fennel seed) that is easy to digest and quick to cook. It has a slightly nutty flavor and is very tasty. Baby basmati is native to Bangladesh and West Bengal.

BLACK (FORBIDDEN) RICE

BOTANICAL NAME ● *Oryza sativa*

SANSKRIT NAME ● *Krishna-vrihi*

Black rice is superbly nutritious, but Ayurveda considers it inferior because it is difficult to digest. Its post-digestive effect is sour. If you have a strong appetite, enjoy black rice occasionally.

SOURCING

- The above varieties are available in health food stores, Asian food stores, or Indian food stores.
- It is best to consume locally grown rice, but that is not possible in all parts of the world.
- The highest quality of rice grown in India comes from the foothills of the Himalayas and other mountains.
- The rule of thumb for selecting rice is to try to source it aged (at least 180 days from the day of harvest) from traditional farmers that have well-maintained seed banks, or purchase the variety that you enjoy and is easy for you to digest.

SEASON

Being tridoshic, rice is a staple suitable to consume all year round.

DIGESTIBILITY

- The different types of rice have gradations of digestibility. Find the ones that work for you. If your gut has a diminished ability to break down starch, you may find that any rice will create a heavy feeling after eating. I've also met people who grew up without much rice in their diet and find it hard to digest as adults. In both cases, either work on improving your digestion or minimize your rice consumption.
- A watery rice soup or porridge (kanji) has been used as a very healing and restorative remedy for recovering after surgery or a severe weakness of the digestive system.
- Refrigerated and then reheated rice is one of the hardest leftovers to digest; it will produce phlegm and bloating.

COOKING TIPS

- Before cooking, gently wash the rice a few times until the water runs clear. This will remove some of the starch and make your cooked grains fluffy.
- Rice types vary in their cooking time, so follow the instructions on the package.
- Soak red or black rice for 30 minutes before cooking to soften it and reduce the cooking time.
- Add an Indian bay leaf or a small piece of cinnamon stick to your rice cooking water—this will help you digest the starch better.
- Always add some fat (i.e., ghee, olive oil, or coconut oil) to your cooked rice, as fat helps break down starch.
- Do not pressure-cook rice because it will break down the grain sugars too fast and cause a blood sugar imbalance. Pressure-cooked rice also tends to create more gas in the gut. (Preparing rice in a rice cooker and keeping it warm there is fine.)
- Cook the rice just before serving. To prevent food poisoning caused by the rapid growth of *Bacillus cereus* spores, do not keep the cooked rice at room temperature for more than 20 minutes. An exception is mixing cooked rice with yogurt—the fermentation from the *Lactobacillus* bacteria prevents the rice from spoiling.

EAT RICE WHEN YOU NEED TO

- add a grounding grain to your meal,
- cool down your body or mind,
- stop loose bowels,
- strengthen your system after illness or surgery, and/or
- build your body.

CAUTION ● The Ayurvedic texts warn us that eating too much rice can cause a lack of glow in our complexion. Oh, well, even the best food when eaten too much can turn against you.

red rice with spinach and nuts

SERVES 2 to 3 ● **SOAK:** 30 minutes ● **PREP:** 5 minutes ● **COOK:** 30 minutes ● **GF, DF** ● **YEAR-ROUND** ●
Photograph on page 64

This is a quick, colorful, and very satisfying dish that could make a light meal on its own.

It is best to use fresh bunched or loose spinach, but packaged triple-washed baby spinach will also work (in this case, it's ready to go straight into the pan). Play with this recipe by substituting thinly cut beet greens, chard, or kale for the spinach or substituting white basmati rice for the red rice.

Red Rice with Spinach and Nuts goes well with a salad or a vegetable soup. You can also serve it with Green Tahini Sauce (page 219), Stuffed Bitter Melon (page 136), Sautéed Bitter Melon (page 135), Cooling Lauki Squash (page 132), and more.

½ cup red rice, rinsed, soaked in water for 30 minutes, and drained

1 teaspoon salt, divided

1 Indian bay leaf

1 tablespoon + ½ teaspoon ghee, olive oil, or coconut oil

1 teaspoon ground coriander

¼ teaspoon ground nutmeg

⅛ teaspoon freshly ground black pepper

6 ounces (about 5½ packed cups) cleaned spinach (stemmed, washed, well drained), roughly chopped

GARNISHES

2 tablespoons pine nuts, cashew pieces, or slivered almonds

2 teaspoons fresh lime juice

FOR VATA OR PITTA BALANCING: Enjoy as is.

FOR KAPHA BALANCING: Reduce the ghee to 2 teaspoons. Add one 1-inch cinnamon stick and 1 small seeded and minced green Indian or Thai chile in Step 3, with the spices.

1. In a 2-quart saucepan, combine 4 cups water, the rice, ½ teaspoon of the salt, and the bay leaf and bring to a boil over high heat. Lower the heat to low and cook, partially covered, for 20 to 30 minutes, until the grains are soft and begin to open up. (Different types of red rice take different times to cook, so look for doneness.) Drain the cooking water, remove the bay leaf, and set aside the rice, covered.

2. In the meantime, make the garnish: Heat ½ teaspoon of the ghee in a small skillet over low heat, and toast the nuts until they turn slightly golden. Set aside.

3. In a medium sauté pan, heat the remaining 1 tablespoon ghee over medium-low heat, add the coriander, nutmeg, black pepper, and the remaining ½ teaspoon salt, and toast until fragrant, about 10 seconds. Add the spinach and sauté until the leaves wilt but remain vibrant green. Add the cooked rice, increase the heat to medium, and, using a large fork or pair of tongs, gently mix and fluff the rice with the spinach for about 5 minutes, to allow the ingredients and flavors to mix well without mashing the grains.

4. Set it aside to let the rice cool down for a minute, then fold in the lime juice. Garnish each serving with the toasted nuts. Serve immediately.

plain basmati rice

SERVES 4 ● **PREP:** 1 minute ● **COOK:** 20 minutes ● **GF, DF** ● **YEAR-ROUND**

This is a base grain recipe that can be used as a "silent" partner in a meal involving dishes with "loud" flavors. Although plain cooked basmati rice is incredibly aromatic, it helps you experience satisfaction in simplicity.

Pair Plain Basmati Rice with any soup, vegetables, or salad. I also use it as part of the filling for Stuffed Cabbage Rolls (page 113) and as the main ingredient in Lime Rice Pilaf (page 65).

1 teaspoon salt

1 cup white basmati rice, washed well and drained

1 tablespoon ghee, coconut oil, or olive oil, divided

1. In a 1- to 2-quart saucepan, bring 2 cups water to a boil and add the salt.

2. Add the rice and 1 teaspoon of the ghee and return to a boil. Cover with a tight-fitting lid, lower the heat to low, and gently simmer for 12 to 15 minutes, until the grains have absorbed the water and are soft but not mushy.

3. Turn off the heat, add the remaining 2 teaspoons ghee, cover, and let the grains set for 5 minutes.

4. Fluff with a fork and serve steamy hot.

Clockwise: Lime Rice Pilaf, Red Rice with Spinach and Nuts, Plain Basmati Rice, Millet Pilaf with Grated Carrots

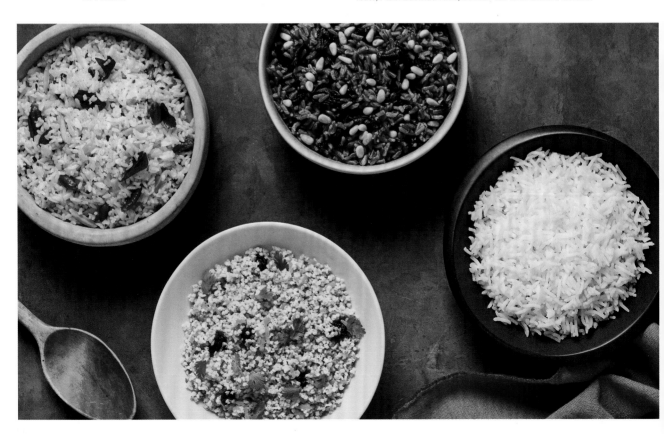

lime rice pilaf

SERVES 2 ● PREP: 5 minutes ● COOK: 7 minutes with already cooked rice ● GF, DF ● YEAR-ROUND

Back in 2015, Vaidya R. K. Mishra and his wife, Melina, visited us in New York City to teach at our Ayurvedic Nutrition and Culinary Training. A couple of hours before they left, they called me and my husband, Prentiss, to their hotel room. There, in the tiny kitchenette, Vaidya showed me how to make two rice recipes. This Lime Rice Pilaf is one of them.

2 teaspoons ghee or coconut oil

¼ teaspoon ground turmeric

¼ teaspoon cumin seeds

1 small green Indian or Thai chile, seeded and minced

1 teaspoon grated fresh ginger

5 fresh curry leaves

¼ teaspoon salt

⅓ cup (1½ ounces) nuts—one or a combination of slivered almonds, cashews, pistachios, halved pecans, halved walnuts, or pine nuts

1½ cups cooked Plain Basmati Rice (page 64, from ½ cup uncooked rice)

1 tablespoon fresh lime juice, or to taste

GARNISH

Fresh cilantro leaves or chopped fresh dill

FOR VATA OR PITTA BALANCING: Omit the chile.

FOR KAPHA BALANCING: Add 1 more small chile and reduce the nuts to ¼ cup. You may also substitute quinoa for the rice.

1. In a 10- to 12-inch skillet, heat the ghee over low heat, and gently toast the turmeric until it darkens a shade and releases its aroma, about 5 seconds. Add the cumin seeds and continue to toast for another 10 seconds, then add the chile, ginger, and curry leaves and toast for 15 seconds more, or until the fresh ingredients crisp up. Add the salt and nuts, increase the heat to medium-low, and toast until the nuts are slightly golden and crisp, 20 to 30 seconds.

2. Add the cooked rice, increase the heat to medium, and stir-fry, using a metal spoon or spatula to toss and stir gently but frequently. In about 5 minutes the rice will become a little drier, less sticky, slightly crispier, and yellow. Try to keep the grains whole and not too mushy.

3. Leave the pilaf uncovered for a couple of minutes to release some of the steam. Add the lime juice and mix with a fork.

4. Garnish with cilantro and serve immediately.

NOTE: If you are allergic to nuts, substitute an equal quantity of shredded coconut or sunflower seeds for the nuts in Step 1. The shredded coconut and sunflower seeds will need only about 10 seconds to turn slightly golden.

WHEAT

There is so much to be said about wheat. Here I will just mention the less known information, in the context of Ayurveda. If you have gluten intolerance, I still encourage you to read this entry because it may help you understand the cause of your intolerance and perhaps give you some ideas of how to possibly reverse it.

Wheat has been grown by human civilizations for thousands of years. Its easy cultivation in almost all parts of the world and its versatility contribute to wheat's integration in the culinary traditions of every culture.

The classical texts of Ayurveda describe three main types of ancient wheat, depending on the geographical areas it was cultivated: *godhuma*, *madhuli*, and *nandhi-mukha*. Each type of wheat grain varies in size and digestibility. I am still trying to identify the Latin botanical names corresponding to the above Sanskrit names, but from the grain description, it seems that *madhuli* comes close to einkorn (a small, easy to digest wheat grain). *Maha-godhuma* (large *godhuma*) is attributed to the ancient wheat grown in the western countries, probably a variety of emmer or spelt.

Ayurveda places wheat in the category of foods that are really good for health (*pathya*) and suitable for daily consumption (*jivana*). The frequency and quantity of consumption will depend on the season, your body constitution and current condition, and your digestive strength.

BOTANICAL NAME ● *Triticum sativum*

SANSKRIT NAME ● *Godhuma, Madhuli, Nandhi-mukha*

AYURVEDIC ATTRIBUTES

TASTE ● sweet, slightly astringent

QUALITIES ● dense, heavy to digest (einkorn is lightest to digest), unctuous

METABOLIC EFFECT ● cooling

POST-DIGESTIVE EFFECT ● sweet

DOSHA EFFECTS ● reduces Vata and Pitta, increases Kapha

HEALING BENEFITS ● gives strength, works as a mild laxative, enhances complexion, acts as an aphrodisiac, has a binding effect in the gut, helps unify fractured bones, supports vitality and longevity

SOURCING

● There are many varieties of wheat today, but if you're health conscious, always select the ancient ones, grown organically: einkorn (the best), Kamut, durum, farro (emmer), and spelt. Use whole flour, ideally freshly milled.

SEASON

● Wheat is a "building" food, and it is most seasonal in cold weather. Avoid eating it when you're congested or trying to lose weight.

DIGESTIBILITY

● Being heavy in nature, wheat calls for strong digestion. Einkorn is the lightest and easiest to digest, and that's why I use it a lot in my recipes.

● Freshly ground flour is much preferred over store-bought flour. Of course, for convenience, most cooks get flour from the grocery store. In that case, pay attention to the packaging date and select the freshest one. The danger of a flour sitting on the shelf (or in your pantry) for a few months is the growth of mold. A lot of people react not only to the gluten but to the mold in flour (and other powders), which is invisible to the naked eye.

- Discard any flour that smells off, stale, musty, or kind of sour, has large clumps, shows signs of mold, or has bugs.
- Always use whole wheat flour. If you need finer flour, sift whole wheat flour to separate its rougher bran.
- Buy small quantities of flour and use it quickly. Refrigerate leftover flour in an airtight container (this will slow down the growth of mold).
- When using einkorn, keep in mind that it is very water soluble; that is, it requires less liquid for making a dough or batter than spelt, emmer, or Kamut. If you're substituting einkorn for spelt, for example, use about a quarter less liquid or increase the einkorn flour by a quarter or a third.

EAT WHEAT WHEN YOU NEED TO

- build weight, strength, and stamina,
- feel satiated and grounded, especially in cold weather, and/or
- satiate your strong appetite.

ayurveda's approach to gluten intolerance

The big digestive issues people began experiencing with wheat started in the mid-1960s, when scientists experimented with intensive hybridization procedures to restructure the wheat proteins in order to create new kinds of wheat that yield more production, enhance water retention, increase pest resilience, and more. The largest seed companies infused the wheat grains with pesticides and insecticides to eliminate the need for spraying field crops and thus reduce farming costs. Unfortunately, the bug killers in the wheat grains we eat also kill the microbiome (the friendly bugs in our gut). The friendly gut bacteria are the first line of defense against "intruders"; they train our immune system how to properly react to pathogens. When our friendly bacteria are weakened or diminished by the chemicals we ingest (through food or pharmaceutical drugs), our immune system goes on high alert. This can lead to autoimmune disorders (including reactions to foods we can no longer digest), chronic inflammation, and more. Inflammation is the entry door to about a hundred serious illnesses.

Although the modern wheat varieties are technically not genetically modified, they are genetically alien. They behave more like a chemical than a food and can lead to tremendous distress in the human digestive tract. To make things worse, the flour of hybrid wheat is stripped of its fiber and essential nutrients and bleached to create different types of white flour for commonly sold breads and pastries. Such denatured wheat products stay in the gut much longer and produce semi-digested sludge (ama) that becomes the breeding ground for disease. When we give our gut the wheat that has been stripped from its essential enzymes and nutrients, how can we expect it to fully break down and assimilate glutenous foods without creating any unpleasant digestive reactions?

Now imagine that you've eaten modern wheat and white flour for many years, and one day you realize that you have a gluten intolerance (or even celiac disease). Yes, we can blame your problem on the modern, alien wheat, and you can switch to a gluten-free diet, but this will only address one side of the issue. The other side is your weakened digestive system and metabolism. You are experiencing reactions because your gut has lost its intelligence to break down gluten—it lingers in your gut for too long, and its nutrients don't fully metabolize into your body tissues. That results in inflammation, skin rashes, aches, pain, and more.

Does the Ayurvedic perspective make sense to you? It made a lot of sense to me ten years ago when I, too, had gluten intolerance (along with chronic inflammation, an autoimmune disorder, and fatigue). Luckily, I am a testimonial of the Ayurveda protocols for successfully treating this chain of conditions by addressing the underlying causes. It is not the purpose of my book to go into these protocols, but if you are interested, I'd suggest that you seek the help of an expert Ayurvedic physician so that you can enjoy eating wholesome bread and cookies again.

sesame crackers two ways: spelt and gluten-free

MAKES about 30 crackers (depending on size) ● **PREP:** 15 minutes ● **BAKE:** about 10 minutes ●
GF OPTION, DF ● **YEAR-ROUND** ● Photograph on pages 195 and 250

We make these crackers at Divya's Kitchen, and I've included them in this book in order to satisfy a frequent request we get from our guests: "Please, can I get the recipe?"

For many of us, crackers are a favorite snack and party food. There are so many options on the market, and it's so much easier to just buy them, but then our bodies have to struggle with the highly processed ingredients and chemical additives found in most store-bought varieties.

My Sesame Crackers are completely clean and wholesome. Children love them! I enjoy them the most when they are very thin. The gluten-free crackers are a bit crunchier, but both options are definitive crowd pleasers. Enjoy them on their own, with dips and sauces, or as a base for hors d'oeuvres. I always take these crackers with me when I'm on the road.

FOR THE SPELT DOUGH

1 cup (125 grams) whole spelt flour, plus more for dusting

1½ tablespoons white sesame seeds or kalonji seeds

½ teaspoon salt

½ teaspoon baking powder

¼ teaspoon black peppercorns, coarsely crushed in a mortar and pestle

2 tablespoons toasted sesame oil or olive oil, plus more for shaping the dough and brushing finished crackers

1½ teaspoons fresh lime juice

1. In a medium bowl, mix the flour, sesame seeds, salt, baking powder, and crushed peppercorns.

2. In a small bowl, whisk the sesame oil, lime juice, and ¼ cup water.

3. Mix the wet ingredients into the dry ingredients, and shape them into a rough dough. (Add more water or flour if necessary.) Knead on a lightly floured surface for about 1 minute, until the dough is soft and smooth. Grease your hands with oil, and shape the dough into a ball.

FOR THE GLUTEN-FREE DOUGH

⅓ cup (40 grams) sorghum flour, plus more for dusting the kneading surface

⅓ cup (36 grams) amaranth flour

⅓ cup (50 grams) buckwheat flour

1 tablespoon arrowroot powder

1 tablespoon white sesame seeds or kalonji seeds

1 teaspoon Italian seasoning or your choice of dried herbs

½ teaspoon salt

¼ teaspoon baking powder

Tiny pinch of asafoetida

2 tablespoons olive oil, plus more for shaping the dough and brushing finished crackers

1. In a medium bowl, mix the sorghum, amaranth, and buckwheat flours, the arrowroot, sesame seeds, Italian seasoning, salt, baking powder, and asafoetida.

2. In a small bowl, whisk ⅓ cup plus 1 tablespoon water with the olive oil. Mix the wet ingredients into the dry ingredients, and shape them into a rough dough. (Add more water or flour if necessary.)

3. Knead on a surface lightly dusted with sorghum flour for about 1 minute, until the dough is soft and smooth. Grease your hands with olive oil, and shape the dough into a ball.

To roll and bake the spelt or gluten-free crackers:

4. Preheat the oven to 400°F. Take out a silicone mat (11½ x 16½ inches), or cut off a piece of parchment paper the same size as your baking sheet (half-size sheet pan is ideal).

5. Place the dough on the mat, and roll it out very thinly (about 1 millimeter). If you're using parchment paper, it might be easier to tape it onto the rolling surface to stabilize it for rolling. You should be able to stretch the dough to fully cover a half-size sheet pan. The thinner you stretch it, the crispier the crackers will be. Prick the dough with a fork. Using a pastry wheel or a knife, cut the crackers into your desired shape (I suggest ½ x 1½-inch rectangles); carefully transfer the mat with crackers to the baking sheet.

6. Bake for 8 minutes and then check every 2 minutes until the crackers turn crisp and pale gold (if they turn dark brown, they will taste bitter). Remove from the oven, and brush the crackers with a thin layer of olive oil.

7. Cool the crackers on the baking sheet. They will keep in an airtight container at room temperature for up to a week.

vegetable bread

SERVES 4 to 6 ● **PREP:** 20 minutes ● **COOK:** 50 minutes ● DF ● **FALL-WINTER**

I think of this bread as a well-to-do focaccia, the Italian flatbread. Well-to-do because it is filled with vegetables and herbs, more opulently than a traditional focaccia. I feel that mixing in more vegetables makes the bread on its own become a sumptuous snack or travel food. The whole spelt flour gives this bread a dark brown base, and the colorful vegetables make it look like a food mosaic.

Pair Vegetable Bread with Basil-Parsley Pesto (page 217) or Ayurvedic "Ketchup" (page 173), and serve it for breakfast or as a side to a soup and salad. At Divya's Kitchen we serve it as an appetizer.

¾ cup diced (⅛-inch) green beans

¾ cup peeled and diced (⅛-inch) carrots

¾ cup diced (⅛-inch) celery

½ cup + 2 tablespoons olive oil, plus more for the pan

2½ cups (285 grams) whole spelt flour

2 teaspoons baking powder

2 teaspoons dried basil

1¼ teaspoons salt (or less if your olives are very salty)

1 teaspoon dried savory or thyme

¾ teaspoon dried oregano

½ teaspoon freshly ground black pepper

Tiny pinch of asafoetida

¼ cup chopped black pitted olives (if too salty, soak them in water overnight, then drain)

1 tablespoon fresh lime juice

1. Heat 1 tablespoon water in an 8-inch skillet over medium-low heat. Add the green beans, carrots, and celery and cook uncovered, stirring occasionally, for 5 minutes, or until the vegetables are half-cooked and vibrant in color. Drain, rinse with cold water, and drain again.

2. Preheat the oven to 350°F. Line a 13 x 9½-inch (quarter-size) sheet pan with parchment paper, and grease it with olive oil.

3. In a medium bowl, combine the flour, baking powder, basil, salt, savory, oregano, pepper, and asafoetida and mix well.

4. In a small bowl, mix together the olive oil, ½ cup + 2 tablespoons water, the olives, lime juice, and cooked vegetables.

5. Fold the wet ingredients into the dry ingredients, using a few strokes to incorporate them into a batter. (Overmixing will make the bread stiff.)

6. Transfer the batter to the prepared sheet pan, and gently press to smooth the top surface. Bake for 40 minutes, or until a toothpick or skewer inserted into the center of the bread comes out clean.

7. Let the bread cool completely in the pan. Cut into your desired shapes. Before serving, warm the pieces, and brush them with a thin layer of olive oil.

Opposite: Vegetable Bread, Basil-Parsley Pesto

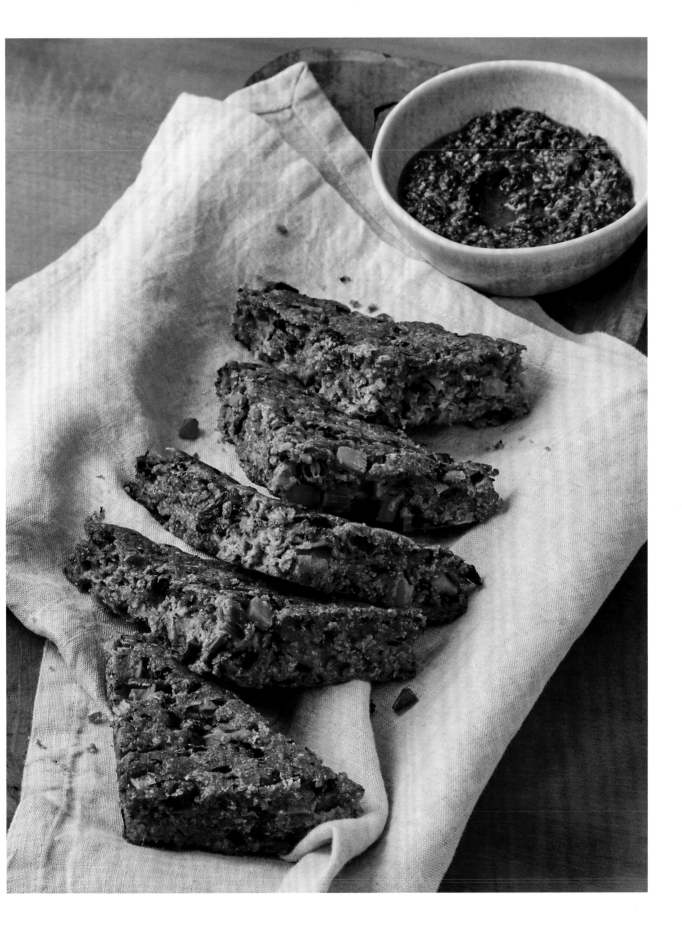

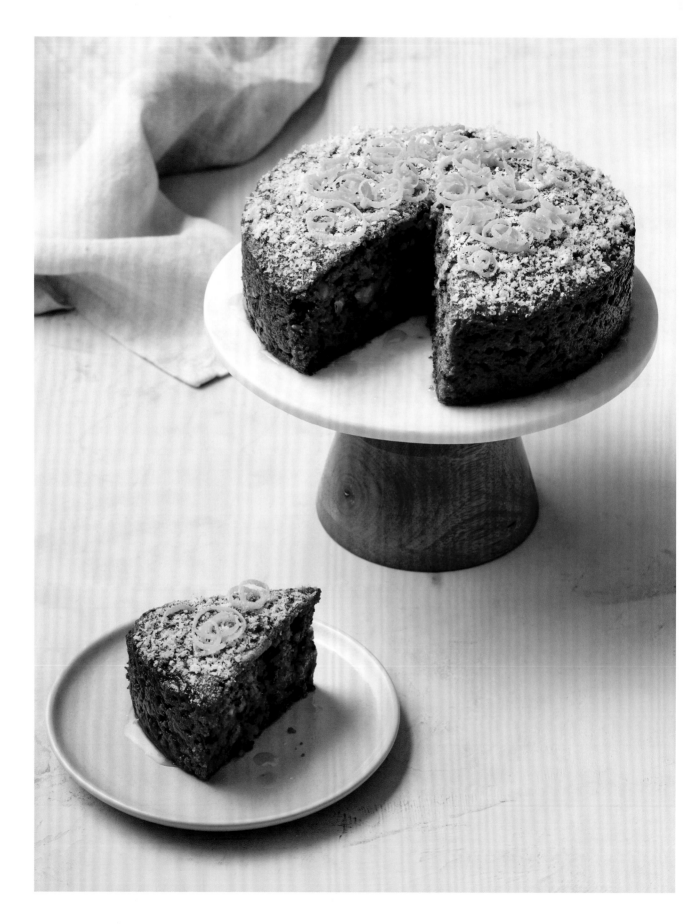

walnut-orange cake with honey syrup

MAKES one 8-inch square or round cake; 9 pieces ● PREP: 30 minutes ● COOK: 30 minutes ●
FALL-WINTER

What is your concept of a healthy cake? Is there such a thing? I say, there is. This recipe is my version of a sugar-free, dairy-free, wholesome pastry, and once you taste it, it might make you want another piece . . . or two.

I love creating healthier versions of favorite desserts, and this recipe is one attempt at doing so. Years ago, my friend Melanie from Greece introduced me to karidopita, a syrupy walnut cake. In her vegan version, she uses olive oil as the fat, dried apricot puree and raw sugar to sweeten the cake, and sugar and honey to sweeten the syrup. In my "Ayurvedized" version, I omit the sugar altogether and add the honey after cooking the flavored syrup. According to Ayurveda, heat turns honey toxic. So don't cook with it.

This cake brings back so many memories of growing up in Bulgaria and loving the Greek and Turkish pastries soaked in sugar-sweet syrup, such as tulumba, kadaifi, baklava, and more. Ah, how good those were! I tasted them again the last time I visited my family in my hometown of Plovdiv, but I was disappointed. The refined white flour and sugar, vegetable oils, and additives not only spoiled the taste but also made the pastries very unhealthy.

If you're a fan of syrupy desserts, try this wholesome option. Succulent, not too sweet, and with an unexpected crunch of walnuts, this cake is satisfying and grounding. Its rustic look reminds one of home. One piece will quiet down your Vata and Pitta and keep your Kapha happy—perfect for the cool season. If your Pitta is too high, replace the honey with maple syrup.

CAKE

½ cup (88 grams) chopped (½-inch pieces) dried apricots

¾ cup boiling hot water

¼ cup olive oil, plus more for greasing the baking dish

2 cups (218 grams) sifted einkorn flour or 1¾ cups (220 grams) sifted spelt flour

1 teaspoon baking powder

1 teaspoon ground cinnamon

¼ teaspoon ground cloves

½ teaspoon baking soda

½ teaspoon fine lime zest

¼ teaspoon salt

½ cup fresh orange juice, from 2 to 3 oranges (before squeezing the oranges, zest their peel for the garnish—see Notes)

1 cup (113 grams) coarsely chopped walnuts

HONEY SYRUP

Peel of ½ orange, thinly sliced

1 cinnamon stick (2¾ inches long)

2 dried apricots, chopped

½ cup raw honey

¼ cup fresh orange juice (strained for pulp)

1 tablespoon fresh lime juice (strained for pulp)

½ teaspoon vanilla extract

CONTINUED

¼ cup toasted and shaved walnuts (see Notes)

Thin orange peel curls (see Notes)

To make the cake:

1. Put the chopped apricots in a blender and pour the boiling water over them. Let them sit for 15 minutes to hydrate. Blend to a smooth puree.

2. Preheat the oven to 350°F. Grease an 8-inch round or square baking dish (a glass Pyrex dish works well) with olive oil.

3. While the apricots are soaking, in a large bowl, whisk together the flour, baking powder, cinnamon, cloves, baking soda, lime zest, and salt.

4. In a medium bowl, whisk together the apricot puree, olive oil, and orange juice.

5. Add the wet mixture to the dry mixture, and stir a few times, until the sticky batter is well incorporated. Fold in the walnuts.

6. Transfer the batter to the greased baking dish. Bake for about 30 minutes, until a toothpick or skewer inserted in the middle of the cake comes out clean. While the cake is baking, prepare the syrup and garnishes. Let the cake completely cool off in the baking dish before transferring it to a cutting board or a serving platter. You may also leave it in the baking dish.

To make the honey syrup:

7. In a small saucepan, combine ¾ cup water, the orange peel, cinnamon stick, and apricots, and bring to a boil over high heat; lower the heat and simmer uncovered for 10 minutes.

8. Remove the orange peel and cinnamon stick, and let the cooked apricots cool down to a warm temperature (not higher than 120°F). Transfer to a blender and blend to a smooth, slightly thick consistency. (If there are any little pieces of fruit left, strain them away.)

9. Pour the blended mixture into a small bowl and whisk in the honey, orange juice, lime juice, and vanilla.

To assemble the cake:

10. Cut the cake into triangle-, square- or diamond-shaped pieces of your desired size.

11. Gradually pour the syrup over the cake, making sure to moisten each of the crevices, edges, and corners. (See Notes if you're not going to serve all cake pieces at once.)

12. Garnish the cake with shaved walnuts and thin curls of orange peel. Serve within 2 hours.

NOTES: If you're not going to serve all the cake pieces at once, pour the syrup and add the garnishes to only the number of pieces you want to serve right now. Refrigerate the rest of the syrup and garnishes until your next serving. Store the remaining cake covered, at room temperature.

To shave the toasted walnuts for garnish, use halved walnuts, and grate them on the small holes of a grater.

To make orange peel curls, use a zester or a julienne peeler to peel off thin strips of orange peel, then soak the strips in a cold-water bath and freeze until you're ready to use them. (It takes at least 45 minutes for the peels to curl.)

on snacking

"What should I do when I'm on a twelve-hour shift at a hospital unit, and I rarely have fifteen minutes to sit down and peacefully eat a full meal? I only get five minutes here and there, enough to pop a snack in my mouth." This question is from my friend Gina, who is a nurse, a mom of three young children, and an Ayurveda enthusiast. She wants to maintain an optimal *agni* by following the ancient guidelines for enjoying full meals at regular times, but her occupation prevents her from eating properly throughout the day. Unfortunately, many of us face her dilemma.

By definition, a snack is supposed to be "a small amount of food" meant to fill the hunger gap between meals, such as the time between an early lunch and a late dinner. However, social norms have encouraged us to pop in our mouths the seemingly casual and harmless bites of chips, pretzels, popcorn, crackers, bars, and cookies—in an almost automatic manner—usually while we entertain ourselves in other ways. Those "small amounts of food" can really add up in a day! If it is true that one-third of the calories that an average American consumes comes from snacks, we face the sad reality that snacking has become a way of eating, and even a way of replacing meals.

Although snacking often gets a bad rap, to say whether it is good or bad isn't so straightforward; it depends on many factors. Nibbling between meals can either support or weaken you and your digestion. First, it is important to understand that food and drink are meant to provide your body with energy, and anytime you ingest something, your body must use energy (a.k.a. work) to digest it. It's helpful to consider this as you make your decision whether to snack: will your snack give you just the right amount of energy for your needs, or will it require excess energy to break down, leaving you feeling more lethargic?

When thinking of intermittent eating, be most attentive to the following situations:

Not eating food when you're hungry (i.e., skipping or delaying meals)—you can alleviate this problem by eating a wholesome snack in a quantity that appeases your hunger, just enough to carry you to your next proper meal. This is what Gina needs to do at work.

Overeating or continuing to eat even though you're full (this includes eating anything before your previous meal has been fully digested); unnecessary snacking—this eating habit can make you sick or overweight.

Do I eat snacks? Absolutely! But I do so as an exception: only when I travel, work peculiar hours, or know that my meal will be delayed. To keep my gut healthy, I don't let snacks creep into my daily eating routine because the set meals of breakfast, lunch, and dinner are meant to not only fuel my body but also mark the milestones of my circadian rhythm. Eating at regular times notifies my organism of the beginning, middle, and end of the day—yet another approach to living in harmony with nature.

Eating a cold, dry, sugary snack on the go can never provide the same nourishment as a hot, substantial meal in a peaceful environment. In situations like Gina's, we sometimes feel like there are no viable options outside of these convenient snack foods. I'm happy to tell you there are healthful ways to address this, and here are some of my ideas: pack some fresh fruit or a thermos with a hot soup or something fresh and warm that you made at home and is easy to eat without extra plates and utensils. Restrain your urge to nibble on the cheap and conveniently packaged ultra-processed snacks you can get from the vending machine or the local deli. And if you opt for purchasing snacks, do not trust the words *healthy* and *all natural* on the wrapper—read the ingredient labels and watch for hydrogenated oils, artificial sweeteners or colors, shortening, and stabilizers; these are the culprits that ever so unnoticeably damage our health.

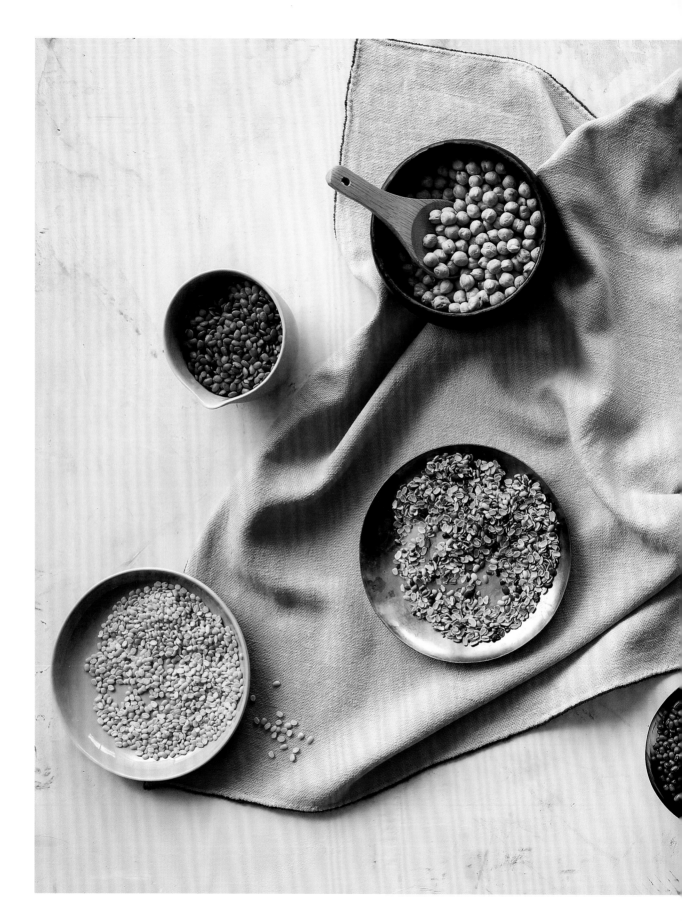

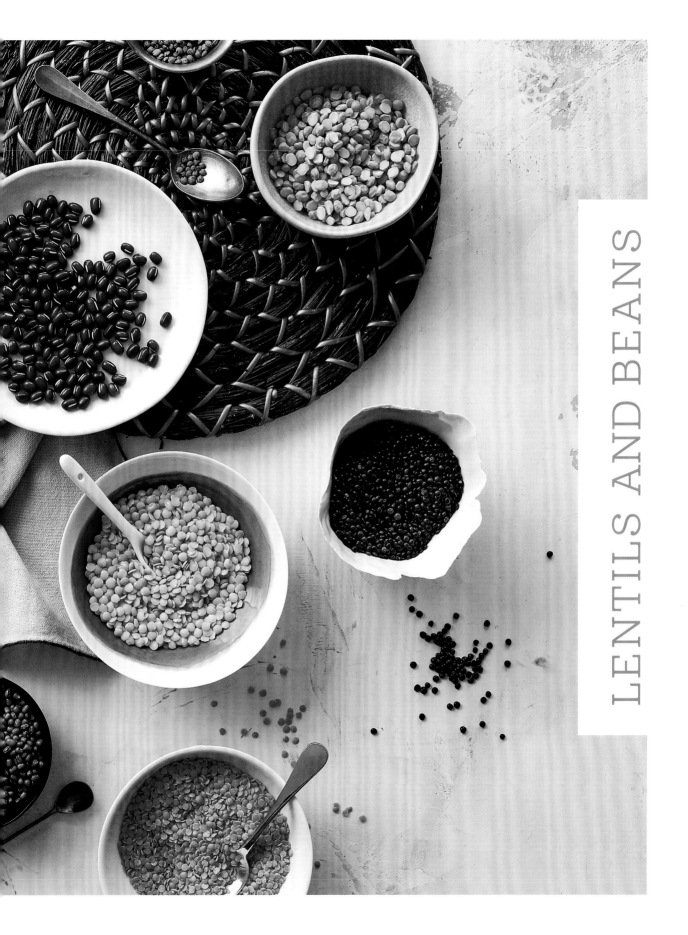

LENTILS AND BEANS

LENTILS AND BEANS

When people ask me to tell them about a traditional Bulgarian dish, I can't help but first think of the white bean soup I grew up with. My father is a master of making it—slow-cooking the soaked beans to a buttery softness while changing the cooking water at least once, then seasoning it with dried Bulgarian savory, fresh parsley, and chopped tomatoes.

Lentils and beans are the dried seeds of legumes and are an important source of protein and fiber, especially in a plant-based diet. They are highly nutritious and contain up to 25 percent protein; however, please select your protein source not just by its nutrition value but mostly by your gut's ability to break it down fully, which allows your system to actually absorb and utilize the protein. Vaidya Mishra once told me that as a vegetarian, I need to eat legumes every day, so I pay close attention to which ones I can digest best. If I feel bloated or too heavy after a meal, I know that those lentils or beans were out of my digestive league.

Different lentils and beans have different attributes. Below I've listed the ones mentioned in the classical Ayurvedic texts that are easiest to digest and recommended for daily or frequent use.

Beware of edamame or soy and its products, including tofu and soy milk, as your source of plant-based protein. Not only is conventional soy genetically modified but unfermented bean products have enzyme inhibitors that obstruct the digestion of protein. Fermented soy products, such as tempeh, miso, soy sauce, or tamari are safer to eat because the fermentation process deactivates the enzyme inhibitors. However, even fermented soy products require strong *agni*, which many people today lack. I've met several people who have experienced dramatic improvements with their gut and skin conditions once they've stopped eating soy. To be on the safe side, I avoid soy completely.

Because most lentils and beans are of astringent taste, they tend to suck up moisture from the body tissues and promote dryness in the body. This drying effect contributes to the clogging and constipating nature of lentils and beans, especially large beans. Soaking the lentils and beans, cooking them in water, and adding a healthy fat will counteract those drying qualities and make them more bioavailable to our organism.

TASTE ● astringent, sweet

QUALITIES ● hard, drying, light (some are heavy) to digest

METABOLIC EFFECT ● cooling or heating

POST-DIGESTIVE EFFECT ● pungent, sweet, or sour

DOSHA EFFECTS ● increase Vata, decrease Pitta and Kapha

HEALING BENEFITS ● provide a good source of plant-based protein, lower high fever, cleanse and nutrify the skin when topically applied as a bean paste

MUNG

BOTANICAL NAME ● *Phaseolus Radiatus*

SANSKRIT NAME ● *Mudga*

Ayurveda declares that among legumes, mung is the best because of its easy digestibility.

Mung is available as the whole bean (green in color), split with the green husk, and shelled and split (yellow in color), which is the lentil-like version of the whole mung bean. The yellow split mung is king in Ayurvedic cooking because it is light and versatile—you can make a soup, kitchari, pancakes, flour for baking, and more.

Mung is of sweet taste, has drying and light qualities, a cooling metabolic effect, and a sweet post-digestive effect. It slightly increases Vata and alleviates Pitta and Kapha. It is good for the eyes, lowers a high fever, and supports the body during disease management or recovery.

RED LENTILS

BOTANICAL NAME ● *Lens Culinaris*

SANSKRIT NAME ● *Masura*

After mung, red lentils are the next best lentil option. They are richer in iron and protein than mung, but still easy to digest. Red lentils are of sweet taste, have drying and light qualities, a cooling metabolic effect, and a sweet post-digestive effect. They increase Vata, alleviate Pitta and Kapha, and, because of their drying effect, can be slightly constipating. They are also useful in reducing a high fever.

KULTHI LENTILS (*HORSE GRAM*)

BOTANICAL NAME ● *Dolichos biflorus*

SANSKRIT NAME ● *Kulattha*

I consider kulthi the most medicinal lentil because of its numerous cleansing benefits. It is of astringent taste, have drying and heavy qualities, a heating metabolic effect, and a sour post-digestive effect.

EAT KULTHI WHEN YOU NEED TO

- balance Kapha and Vata (or increase Pitta),
- break down kidney stones or gallstones,
- dissolve growths,
- reduce joint inflammation,
- alleviate asthma,
- lose fat,
- lower a high fever,
- purge worms,
- decongest or dry a cough,
- cleanse your body in general, and/or
- eliminate hemorrhoids.

CAUTION ● Because of its strong effects, do not eat kulthi more than two to three times per week, unless supervised by an Ayurvedic practitioner.

CHICKPEAS

BOTANICAL NAME ● *Cicer Arietinum Linn.*

SANSKRIT NAME ● *Chanaka*

The chickpea is of astringent taste; it has drying, rough, and heavy to digest qualities, a cooling metabolic effect, and a pungent post-digestive effect. It balances Pitta and Kapha, and increases Vata, and thus it can cause constipation. It is useful in building the body and lowering a high fever. Among the different species of chickpea, the more common are the garbanzo beans (popular in the West) and chana dal, which is the split and shelled version of the black chickpea variety and is the easiest to digest.

CONTINUED

SOURCING

- Lentils and beans are lighter to digest when they're used within one year after harvesting and drying them. The older they get, the longer they take to cook. It's best to purchase them organic, from the bulk section of a grocery store, as the high consumer purchase in bulk ensures ingredient freshness. Indian grocery stores carry the native varieties of mung, red lentils, kulthi, and chana dal.

SEASON

- You can enjoy lentils and beans all year round. I recommend heavier whole beans more in the winter (when digestion is stronger), cooked sprouted beans in the spring, and lighter split lentils in the summer and early fall (although they are balancing all year round).

DIGESTIBILITY

- For a lot of people, beans mean bloating and gas. Because of their airy nature and astringent taste, they are already challenging to the stomach. The larger the bean and the harder its skin, the more dryness it creates in the physical channels, thus increasing the probability of clogged channels—large garbanzo, red kidney, lima, peas, and pinto are some examples of large beans. In Shaka Vansiya Ayurveda, we advise eating larger beans only occasionally and if you are physically active and have a strong appetite. If your digestion is irregular or sluggish, the partially digested beans will likely create blockages and acidic buildup in your gut.

- The easiest-to-digest are split or whole lentils and small beans, such as the varieties mentioned above. Many modern varieties also fall in that group: adzuki, green French lentils, black (a.k.a. beluga) lentils, brown lentils, and more.

- Someone who is lectin intolerant will have difficulty digesting lentils. Properly cooking them significantly improves the lectin breakdown, which is why it is important to cook your lentils and not eat them raw. Raw, sprouted beans are very airy and irritating to the gut and therefore are not recommended for daily use.

- Avoid eating leftover cooked lentils (and canned beans for that matter), as they are hard to digest and will give you a lot of gas.

COOKING TIPS

- Soak whole beans in boiling hot water overnight and lentils for at least 30 minutes—this supports lectin digestion and shortens cooking time.

- To wash lentils, place them in a mesh strainer with a bowl underneath. Fill up the bowl with water, and gently rub the lentils until the water is cloudy. Lift the strainer with lentils, discard the starchy water, then fill up the bowl again and repeat this washing process until the water runs more or less clear.

- Toast the soaked, rinsed, and well-drained lentils in ghee or oil for about 10 minutes over low heat, until they dry up. Vaidya R. K. Mishra told me that this cooking method improves the digestion of lectins.

- Pressure-cooking, although convenient, is not ideal because it breaks down the carbohydrates too fast, making them harder to properly absorb and transform in the body. I pressure-cook beans only as a last resort if I'm pressed for time.

- Add salt toward the end of cooking, especially for whole beans. Salt's minerals harden the water and the beans while cooking.

- The flour of chana or mung dal mixed with water into a paste has been used for centuries as a "soap" to clean and nutrify the skin. See my skin cleanser recipes on pages 54, 93, and 192 for ways to do that.

ENJOY WELL-COOKED LENTILS AND BEANS DAILY OR OCCASIONALLY WHEN YOU NEED TO

- increase your fiber intake,
- incorporate an easy-to-digest, plant-based protein into your diet,
- have gentle nourishment while recovering from an acute illness or surgery (make a light broth),
- strengthen your muscles and body in general,
- stop loose bowels,
- recover from a high fever, and/or
- do a gentle cleansing (especially with kulthi lentils).

kulthi lentil stew, puerto rican style

SERVES 4 ● SOAK: at least 8 hours or overnight ● PREP: 20 minutes ● COOK: about 75 minutes ● GF, DF ●
FALL-WINTER-SPRING

This recipe makes me so proud. It was created by Maria Torres as her final project at the first Ayurvedic Nutrition and Culinary Training we facilitated in 2015-16. At the beginning of the program, Maria told me that she didn't have the confidence to even boil water, let alone cook Ayurvedic food. Closer to her graduation, Maria demonstrated her outstanding progress by presenting this stew recipe of complex flavors that is most delicious and satiating. It also delivers the notable healing benefits of kulthi, and it tastes so good, you will forget that it's healthy!

Maria shares why she created this recipe: "I recently made a kitchari with kulthi lentils for my Puerto Rican family, and they were not impressed. If anything, they felt sorry for me. I decided to create an Ayurvedic version of a traditional Puerto Rican bean stew (that resembles the effect of kitchari) with familiar flavors but unexpected ingredients. Maintaining the traditional sofrito flavors without garlic, onion, and green pepper was a challenge. I used alternatives like asafoetida, capers, black pepper, black cardamom, olives, and saffron."

Serve Kulthi Lentil Stew, Puerto Rican Style with Plain Basmati Rice (page 64). It will also go well with a side salad or cooked vegetables. Due to its powerful cleansing properties, enjoy it not more than twice a week.

½ cup kulthi lentils, soaked in hot water at least 8 hours overnight, rinsed, and drained

½ cup red lentils, washed, soaked in water for 25 minutes, and drained

1 cup peeled and diced (½-inch) taro root or yautia

1 cup peeled and diced (½-inch) carrots

2 tablespoons olive oil or ghee

1½ teaspoons salt, or to taste (olives and capers will add saltiness)

¼ cup chopped fresh cilantro

1 tablespoon peeled and grated fresh ginger

1 tablespoon fresh sweet tamarind pulp, broken into small chunks, or 2 tablespoons Ayurvedic "Ketchup" (page 173)

3 pitted green olives, finely diced (optional)

1 teaspoon capers, rinsed (optional)

1 teaspoon ground coriander

1 teaspoon ground cumin

1 small green Indian or Thai chile, seeded and minced

½ teaspoon ground turmeric

½ teaspoon dried oregano

2 black cardamom pods

2 bay leaves

Pinch of saffron

Tiny pinch of asafoetida

¼ cup chopped (½-inch long) green beans or asparagus

¼ teaspoon freshly ground black pepper

GARNISHES

Olive oil

¼ cup fresh cilantro leaves

Avocado wedges

CONTINUED

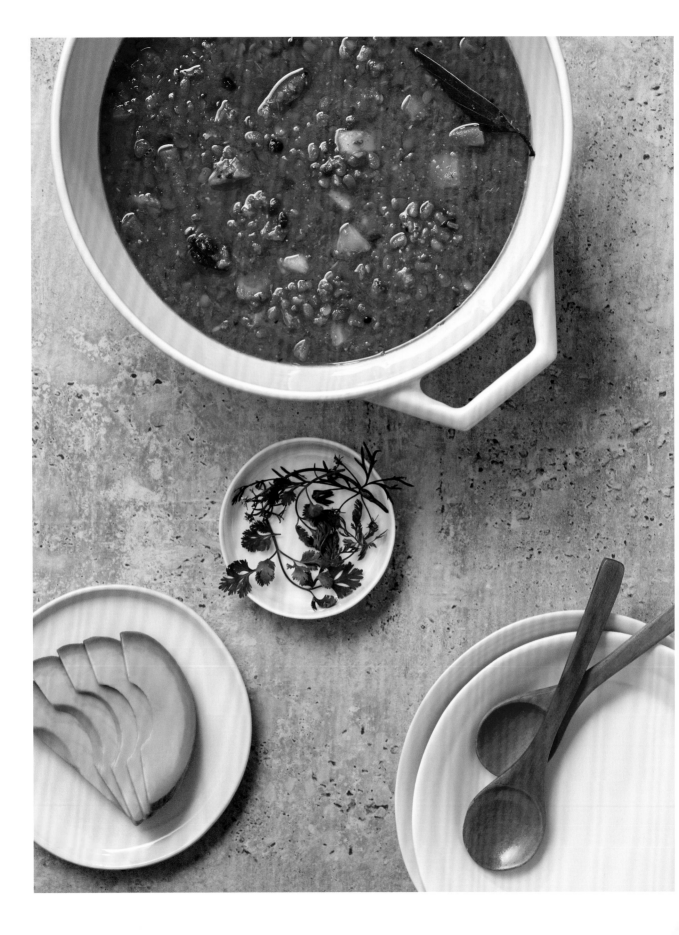

FOR VATA BALANCING: Enjoy as is.

FOR PITTA BALANCING: Omit the olives, capers, black pepper, and tamarind or Ayurvedic "Ketchup." Add 1 extra teaspoon ground coriander in Step 2.

FOR KAPHA BALANCING: Add 1 more green chile in Step 2.

1. In a small saucepan, cover the kulthi lentils with about 1 inch water and bring to a boil over high heat. Lower the heat and cook covered for 50 minutes. The kulthi should be much softer but not yet done. Keep in mind that this lentil is very hard and will not break down like red lentils do; it will keep its shape and be a little crunchy even when fully cooked.

2. Meanwhile, pour 2 cups water into a 3-quart saucepan and turn the heat to medium. Add the red lentils, taro root, carrots, olive oil, and salt. Simmer covered for 5 minutes, then add the cilantro, ginger, tamarind, olives and capers, the coriander, cumin, chile, turmeric, oregano, black cardamom, bay leaves, saffron, and asafoetida. Cover, lower the heat to medium-low, and simmer for 10 minutes.

3. Add the green beans and cooked kulthi with enough of its cooking liquid to keep a medium-thick stew consistency. Cover and continue to simmer for about 25 minutes, stirring occasionally, until the vegetables and kulthi are soft and the stew is creamy.

4. Turn off the heat. Remove and discard the cardamom pods and bay leaves. Stir in the black pepper and check if you need to adjust the salt.

5. For a genuine Puerto Rican finish, garnish each bowl a drizzle of olive oil and some cilantro leaves. Serve hot with avocado wedges on the side.

Opposite: Kulthi Lentil Stew, Puerto Rican Style

kulthi tea

MAKES 1 cup ● PREP: 5 minutes ● GF, DF ● YEAR-ROUND

I learned this very medicinal tea from Dr. Marianne Teitelbaum's book *Healing the Thyroid with Ayurveda* (Healing Arts Press, 2019). She recommends it as the best natural remedy for safely breaking down gallstones and kidney stones, especially if they are small. This tea is good to take daily for three to six months, after which you can visit a doctor to reevaluate your condition. Do not use it if you're pregnant or nursing.

2 tablespoons kulthi lentils, rinsed and drained
1 cup boiling hot filtered or spring water

1. Place the kulthi in a small bowl or large mug and pour in the boiling hot water. Cover and let it steep on the counter overnight.

2. The next morning, drain and reserve both the lentils and water in separate containers. Sip the water, warming it up, if you like. Cover the lentils with more water, and refrigerate.

3. That night, strain the lentils and repeat Step 1 and then Step 2 the next morning.

4. Repeat Steps 1 to 3 for a third time with the same lentils. After that, you could cook them into a soup (see Note).

5. On the evening of the third day, repeat the recipe, starting with a fresh batch of soaked lentils.

NOTE: On the third day, cook the lentils with 1 cup mixed chopped asparagus, daikon radish, and taro root (for an inspiration, see Kulthi Lentil Stew, Puerto Rican Style, page 81).

adzuki bean and red lentil patties

MAKES ten 2½-inch patties ● SOAK: 8 hours or overnight ● PREP: 15 minutes ● COOK: about 90 minutes ●
GF, DF ● FALL-WINTER-SPRING

As part of our Ayurvedic Nutrition and Culinary Training, Annie Mymokhod created this tasty recipe for her final project. When I first met Annie's family of two well-behaved teenagers and her kind and supportive husband, I was astonished by their love for healthy home-cooked food and family meals. Annie is very resourceful in creating appealing vegetarian versions of common "American" foods, keeping the familiar names yet following the Ayurvedic principles of compatibility and preparation. In her words, "My kids were my toughest judges, and when I presented them with this version of a veggie burger, they were pleasantly surprised at how good it tasted! These burgers became an instant success with my family, and I am excited to share this recipe with you."

This recipe may seem time-consuming, but you could stage the steps over a few hours, have the mix ready, and panfry right before mealtime.

Adzuki Bean and Red Lentil Patties go well with a sauce, such as Ayurvedic "Ketchup" (page 173), Green Tahini Sauce (page 219), or Roasted Carrot Tahini Sauce (page 148), and a nice salad on the side. You could also use them as party food by shaping smaller patties (1½ to 2 inches in diameter), topping them with a sauce, and arranging them on a platter or using them in a slider sandwich. You can even prepare them as a travel food.

½ cup adzuki beans, soaked in water at least 8 hours or overnight, drained, and rinsed

½ cup red lentils, washed and drained

1 small red beet, peeled and very thinly sliced (about ½ cup)

1 teaspoon coriander seeds

½ teaspoon cumin seeds

¼ teaspoon black peppercorns

⅛ teaspoon asafoetida

2 tablespoons ghee or olive oil

2 teaspoons grated fresh ginger

1 medium zucchini, cut into ¼-inch-thick half-moons (1½ to 2 cups)

1 cup quinoa flakes (or a little more if the batter is too soft)

1 tablespoon finely chopped fresh flat-leaf parsley

1 tablespoon finely chopped fresh dill

1 tablespoon fresh lime juice

1¼ teaspoons salt

About ¼ cup ghee or coconut oil for panfrying

GARNISHES

2 avocados, sliced into thin wedges (optional)

A few fresh cilantro leaves

FOR VATA BALANCING: Enjoy as is.

FOR PITTA BALANCING: Omit or reduce the asafoetida and black pepper.

CONTINUED

Opposite: Adzuki Bean and Red Lentil Patties, Steamed Kale Salad, Green Tahini Sauce, Ayurvedic "Ketchup"

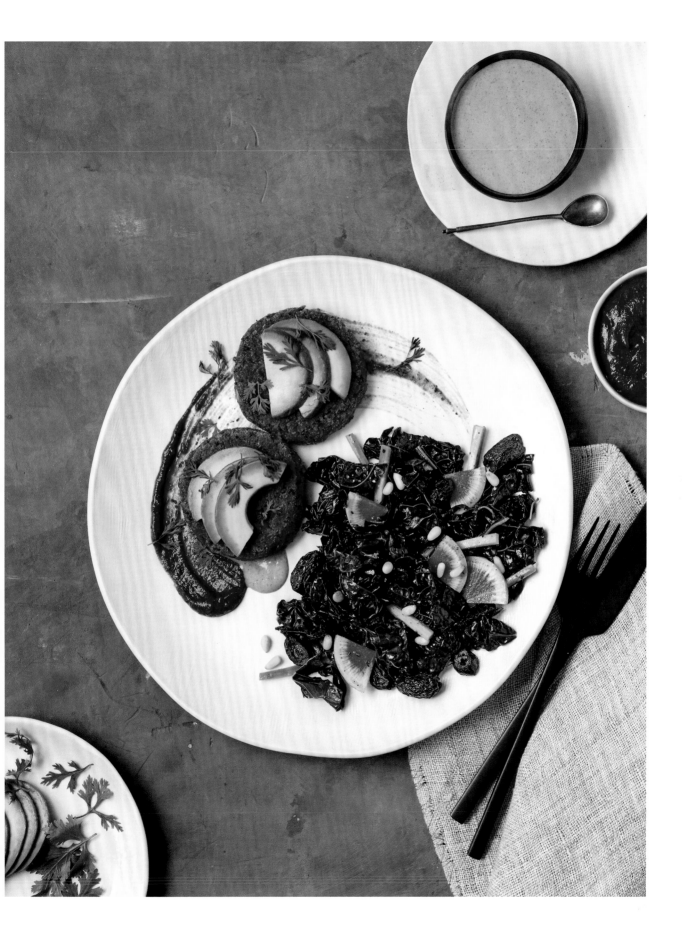

1. Place the adzuki beans in a small saucepan, add enough water to cover them by 1 inch, and bring to a boil over high heat. Cover with a tight-fitting lid, lower the heat to low, and simmer for about 1 hour, until the beans are tender and fully cooked. Drain and set aside to cool.

2. Meanwhile, place the red lentils and beets in another small saucepan and add 1½ cups water. Bring to a boil over high heat. Cover with a tight-fitting lid, lower the heat to low, and simmer for about 10 minutes, until the lentils start to break down and most of the water has been absorbed. Drain and set aside to cool, uncovered.

3. Using a spice grinder, grind the coriander seeds, cumin seeds, peppercorns, and asafoetida to a fine powder.

4. Heat the ghee in a medium skillet over medium-low heat. Add the ginger and spice blend; toast for about 10 seconds, then stir in the zucchini. Sauté for 5 minutes, or until the zucchini softens and mixes well with the spices. Set aside uncovered.

5. To make the patty mixture: Add the cooked adzuki beans, red lentils and beets, spiced zucchini, quinoa flakes, parsley, dill, lime juice, and salt to a food processor. Pulse for 1 to 2 minutes, until all the ingredients are mixed well. The mixture should be fairly soft but not runny. If it is runny, add a little more quinoa flakes to firm it up. Keep in mind that the mixture will continue to thicken as it rests on the counter or in the refrigerator.

6. Heat a large cast-iron griddle over medium heat; brush the surface of the pan with a thin layer of ghee. Fill a ¼-cup measuring cup or scoop with the patty mixture, quickly flop it onto the hot skillet, and shape it into a burger patty. Repeat with the remaining patty mixture, fitting 3 or 4 patties on the griddle at a time and adding more ghee as needed. Watch the ghee to make sure it does not smoke; if it does, lower the heat or turn it off for a few seconds to cool down the pan a bit. Panfry the patties until their bottom sides turn golden and crusty, 2 to 3 minutes. Brush the top, uncooked sides with a thin layer of ghee, then flip them and cook until their second sides are golden and firm, another 1 to 2 minutes. The patties should be soft yet holding together. They will firm up as they cool down.

7. Transfer the cooked patties onto a platter (do not stack them to ensure they keep their crispy exterior). Serve hot, with a side of sliced avocado, some cilantro leaves, and a sauce.

red lentil and celery root soup

SERVES 4 ● SOAK: 30 minutes ● PREP: 10 minutes ● COOK: 35 minutes ● GF, DF ● FALL-WINTER-SPRING

This was one of the first recipes I learned from Vaidya Mishra. He used it as an example of preparing an easy-to-digest protein while stressing that it is not so much about how many grams of protein you take in but how well you can break down and assimilate the protein molecules. Spices play a big role in this assimilation process. The flavor combinations of the earthy red lentils, anise-sweet celery root, and fragrant masala produce an enchanting blend for aromatherapy in your kitchen.

Celery root (a.k.a. celeriac, celery knob) is a bit messy to work with—I handle its knobbiness and dirt-filled crevices by peeling it with a knife. It's worth the effort, though, as this fall/winter vegetable nourishes us with potassium and phosphorus and helps us ground our airy energies. Cooked with red lentils as I show with this recipe, celery root contributes to an enjoyable, mineral-rich soup that is very balancing during the cold season.

1 cup red lentils, soaked in water for 30 minutes, rinsed well, and drained

1 small celery root, peeled and diced into ¼-inch pieces (about 1 cup)

2 tablespoons ghee or olive oil, divided

1½ teaspoons salt

½ teaspoon cumin seeds

¼ teaspoon ground turmeric

6 fresh curry leaves

1 small green Indian or Thai chile, seeded and minced

½ teaspoon Warming Masala (page 233)

1 tablespoon + 1 teaspoon fresh lime juice, or to taste

GARNISHES

Olive oil

2 tablespoons minced fresh dill or whole cilantro leaves

FOR VATA BALANCING: Enjoy as is.

FOR PITTA BALANCING: Omit the green chile. Add 1 teaspoon ground fennel with the spices in Step 1.

FOR KAPHA BALANCING: Reduce the ghee or olive oil to 1 tablespoon (use half of it in Step 1 and the rest in Step 2), and double the amount of the green chile and Warming Masala.

1. Combine the red lentils with 4 cups water in a heavy 3-quart saucepan. Bring to a full boil over high heat, stirring occasionally and removing any froth from the surface. Add the celery root, 1 tablespoon of the ghee, the salt, cumin seeds, turmeric, curry leaves, and chile. Once the soup is boiling again, lower the heat to medium-low and cover. Simmer gently until the celery root is tender and the lentils are starting to break apart, about 30 minutes, stirring occasionally to keep the ingredients from sticking to the bottom of the pan. Turn off the heat.

2. Heat the remaining 1 tablespoon ghee in a small skillet or a metal measuring cup over low heat. Add the Warming Masala and toast for 5 seconds. Pour into the soup, and immediately cover to allow the spice blend to steep for 1 minute.

3. Stir in the lime juice. Serve hot, garnishing each individual bowl with a drizzle of olive oil and dill.

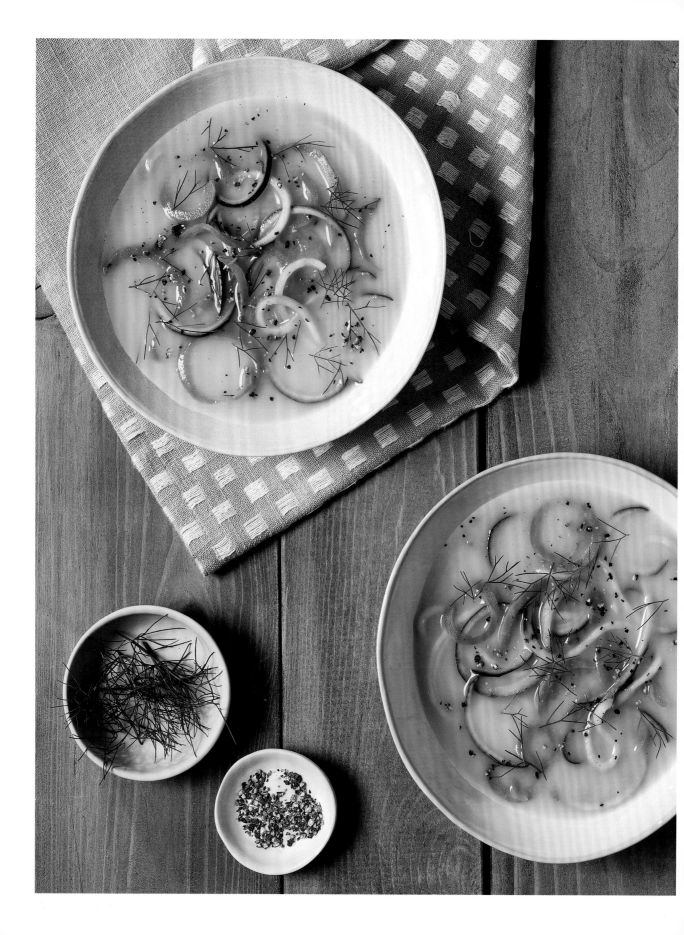

dill-mung soup
with vegetable noodles

SERVES 3 to 4 ● SOAK: 30 minutes ● PREP: 15 minutes ● COOK: 30 minutes ● GF, DF ● SUMMER-FALL

Think of this soup as a vegetarian counterpart to a restorative and comforting chicken noodle soup. It is so delicate, nourishing, and satisfying—it will make you feel stronger in no time.

This is a variation of a recipe by my late mentor Yamuna Devi. She was a true master of food and flavor and taught me so much about cooking with a loving intention. I love how she made mung dal more playful by having noodled vegetables swim in it. The thinly creamed mung provides a smooth base for the colorful vegetable noodles to stand out and make a statement (or a splash if you eat them too fast!). Of course, you can also slice the vegetables if you're cooking in a hurry, but try this recipe as it is written below at least once. Its looks won't disappoint you.

Dill-Mung Soup with Vegetable Noodles has a thin broth-like consistency and subtle, calming flavors. It can make a light summer dinner or lunch with a grain dish such as Plain Basmati Rice (page 64) or Gluten-Free Paratha Flatbread (page 56) or with Steamed Kale Salad (page 109).

4 cups Quick Vegetable Broth (page 143)

½ cup yellow split mung dal, rinsed, soaked in water for 30 minutes, and drained

2 teaspoons ghee

2 teaspoons slivered fresh ginger

4 fresh curry leaves

1 teaspoon ground fennel

1 teaspoon salt

3 ounces carrot noodles (see Note), from 1 medium carrot (1½ cups loosely packed)

5 ounces zucchini noodles (see Note), from 1 medium zucchini (2 cups loosely packed)

1 tablespoon fresh lime juice

1½ teaspoons minced fresh dill

GARNISHES

Olive oil

Freshly ground black pepper

1½ teaspoons minced fresh dill

FOR VATA OR PITTA BALANCING: Enjoy as is.

FOR KAPHA BALANCING: Add 1 seeded and minced green Indian or Thai chile with the spices in Step 1.

1. In a 4-quart pot, combine the broth and mung dal and bring to a boil over medium-high heat. Skim the froth from the boiling surface, then add the ghee, ginger, curry leaves, fennel, and salt. Bring to a boil again, then lower the heat to low and simmer covered for about 20 minutes, until the dal is cooked and starts to break apart. Turn off the heat and set aside the pot uncovered to allow the soup to cool down a bit.

CONTINUED

2. Using a blender, blend the soup to a very smooth consistency, then return it to the pot. Alternatively, you can run the cooked dal through a fine-mesh strainer, pressing the solids to extract as much creaminess from them as possible.

3. Add 1 cup water to the mung soup, and bring it to a gentle boil over medium heat. Add the carrot noodles, cover, lower the heat to low, and simmer for 3 minutes. Add the zucchini noodles and continue to simmer uncovered for another minute, or until the vegetables are soft but have a slight crunch, not too hard or mushy.

4. Turn off the heat and remove the lid. When the soup cools a bit, stir in the lime juice and dill. Garnish each bowl a drizzle of olive oil, black pepper, and dill. Serve hot and, depending on the length of your noodles, offer spoons or chopsticks as eating utensils.

NOTES: Ideas for making vegetable noodles:

If you have a spiralizer, use the spaghetti blade. Cut the noodles short or leave them longer, depending on what eating utensils you want to serve the soup with (spoons for shorter noodles or chopsticks for longer ones).

If you don't have a spiralizer, make fettuccine-like flat noodles by shaving the carrot and zucchini with a peeler—keep turning the vegetable after each shave to keep the noodles narrow. You can also cut the shaved pieces lengthwise to make the noodles even thinner.

You can also use the julienne blade of a mandoline.

how to sprout mung beans

MAKES 2 cups sprouts SOAK: 8 hours or overnight ● PREP: 3 minutes ● SPROUT: 6 to 8 hours ● GF, DF ● SPRING

Making your own bean sprouts might be intimidating, but it is actually quite easy. For guaranteed success, use a sprouting jar or another sprouting device rather than a strainer.

By mung sprouts, I mean home-made sprouted beans with short tails. I don't mean the long and crunchy mung sprouts commonly sold in grocery stores and used in Asian-style cuisines. The longer the sprouted tails, the starchier and heavier the beans.

1 cup whole mung beans, ideally organic because they sprout better

1. Soak the mung beans in cold water, on the counter, for at least 8 hours or overnight.

2. Strain and rinse the soaked beans. Place them in a sprouting container or a covered mesh strainer with a bowl underneath. Keep the beans moist and in darkness while they sprout. The time for the shoots to grow 2 to 3 millimeters varies, but it usually takes 6 to 8 hours—check on them every few hours.

3. Rinse the mung bean sprouts and drain them well before using them. You can store them refrigerated in an airtight container for up to three days—always sort the sprouts to remove the hard, unsprouted beans, and rinse and drain them before use.

Opposite: Sautéed Mung Sprouts

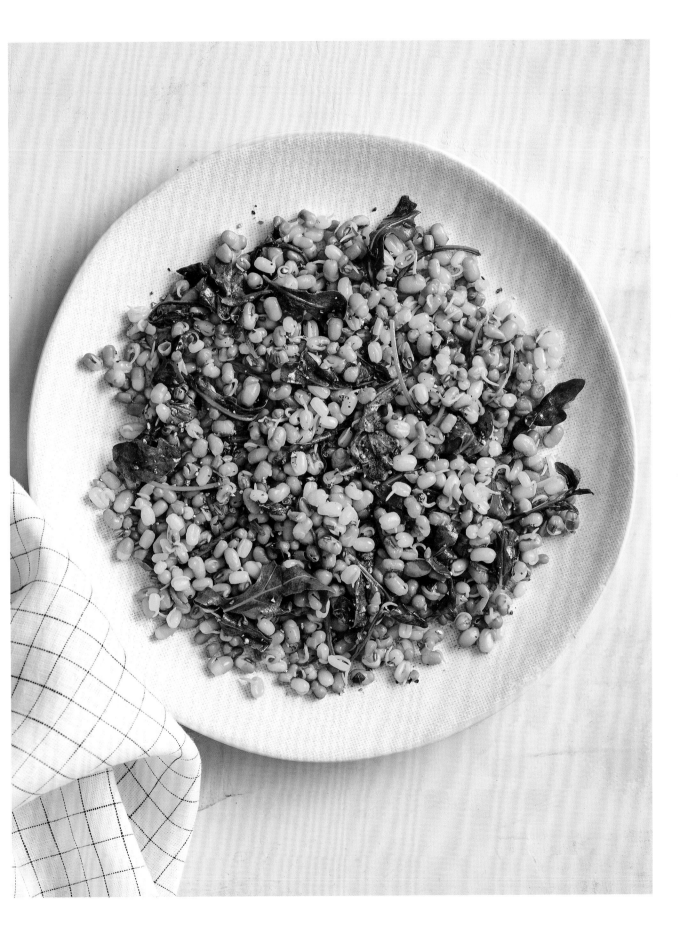

sautéed mung sprouts

SERVES 2 to 4 ● PREP: about 15 minutes (with already made sprouts) ● COOK: 5 minutes ● GF, DF ● SPRING

Sprouted seeds, grains, and beans are most seasonal during spring, when nature begins to "sprout" back to life. Sprouting activates growth and increases the nutritional value and digestibility of a food, but don't go too crazy with sprouts, especially if you are a Vata type, because they are very airy by nature. To minimize the gas-producing quality of bean sprouts, Ayurveda recommends that we lightly sauté them with warming spices.

My husband, Prentiss, and I love eating this dish for breakfast during the spring months because it is filling but light. Use this recipe as a base for countless variations (see some suggestions below). You can also have it as a side dish for lunch.

2 cups fresh mung sprouts (page 90)

2 tablespoons olive oil

1 small green Indian or Thai chile, seeded and minced (optional)

½ teaspoon ground turmeric

½ teaspoon salt

Tiny pinch of asafoetida

2 cups loosely packed baby arugula, sunflower greens, pea shoots, or any other small leafy greens

1 tablespoon fresh lime juice

Freshly ground black pepper

FOR VATA BALANCING: Replace the chile with 1 tablespoon thinly slivered fresh ginger.

FOR PITTA BALANCING: Omit the green chile and asafoetida. Add 1 teaspoon ground fennel with the spices in Step 2.

FOR KAPHA BALANCING: Enjoy as is.

1. Spread the mung sprouts on a tray and sort through them and remove any hard, unsprouted beans (those are really hard and could break a tooth). Rinse and drain well.

2. In a medium sauté pan, heat the olive oil over low heat, add the chile, turmeric, salt, and asafoetida, then stir in the sprouts. Increase the heat to medium-low and sauté for about 10 minutes, until the sprouts become soft and succulent. If the sprouts start to dry too fast, turn down the heat and splash in a little more water.

3. Turn off the heat, add the greens, and toss quickly until the greens are wilted. Mix in the lime juice and garnish with black pepper. Serve warm.

VARIATION: Add 1 cup finely diced carrots with the sprouts in Step 2. Add diced red radishes and celery with the greens in Step 3. (You might have to add a bit more water to keep the dish moist.) Adjust the salt and pepper to taste.

care for sensitive skin

Sensitive skin is common for people with a Pitta constitution, but regardless of your constitution, it can also be a sign of a high Pitta imbalance in your skin. Prolonged exposure to strong sunlight, working in a very hot environment, topical applications of chemical substances, an overheated liver, and more could cause sensitive skin. If you're experiencing redness, a rash, burning, blisters, intolerance to touch, or acne, you have sensitive skin, and it needs to be cooled and calmed. Try the recipes below, and also check out my recommendations for external use of aloe vera on page 214.

You'll find cleanser recipes for oily skin on page 54 and for dry skin on page 192.

skin cleansing powder for sensitive skin

This is another recipe inspired by Dr. Pratima Raichur. This natural cleanser and gentle exfoliator is inexpensive and quick to make, and it will keep your skin bright and leave your face feeling clean, fresh, and toned without any dryness. Use it daily, in the morning and evening.

3 tablespoons almond meal (or grind 10 to 12 almonds to a fine powder)

2 tablespoons chickpea flour

1 teaspoon ground dried rose petals

½ ounce liquid coconut oil or sweet almond oil, ideally in a small bottle with a dropper

TO MAKE: Using a mortar and pestle, mix the almond meal, chickpea flour, and rose powder well. Transfer to a small airtight jar and store in the vanity cabinet of your bathroom. Use within ten days.

TO USE: Remove any makeup (a few drops of sweet almond oil on a cotton ball works great for this).

In your palm, place about ½ teaspoon of the cleansing powder, 2 to 3 drops of coconut oil, and a few drops of rose water or tap water, enough to make a spreadable paste.

Rub the paste on your two palms (like soap), and gently massage it all over your face and neck in an upward and outward direction. Do not scrub hard. Rinse well with warm (not hot) water, and wipe with a damp washcloth. Follow with a facial mask, or let your skin air dry naturally before applying a nourishing oil and/or a moisturizer.

probiotic mask for sensitive skin

This mask helps restore the friendly bacteria in the skin. Apply up to three times per week, after cleaning your face.

1 tablespoon chickpea flour

2 teaspoons plain whole yogurt (or enough to make a paste)

¼ teaspoon ground manjishtha

1 drop of sandalwood, rose, or lavender essential oil (optional)

TO MAKE: Mix all the ingredients in a tiny bowl.

TO USE: Apply the mixture on your face, and leave on the mask for 10 minutes. Rinse well with warm water, and wipe with a damp washcloth. Follow with a nourishing oil and/or a moisturizer.

simple kitchari

SERVES 4 ● SOAK: 30 to 60 minutes ● PREP: 10 minutes ● COOK: about 40 minutes ● GF, DF ●
YEAR-ROUND

If you are looking for healthy comfort food, kitchari is your answer. This creamy, light, and soothing one-pot meal is the Ayurveda superstar—easy to make, inexpensive, delicious, and teeming with health benefits. It is not only nourishing but also cleansing and assists in resetting your digestive system and recovering from illness or fatigue. You can do a kitchari "cleanse" as a way to detox your body and mind, in which you eat nothing but kitchari for three to five days. Whether you're trying to lighten up your body or need to prepare a complete meal in forty minutes, kitchari is there for you, any day of the year. (Admittedly, I've eaten a lot of kitchari during my busy schedule of writing this book!)

I'm proud to say that Simple Kitchari was published twice in *Bon Appétit*'s *Healthyish* magazine. It goes well with Green Tahini Sauce (page 219) or Ayurvedic "Ketchup" (page 173). It also pairs well with a salad or sautéed leafy greens.

½ cup yellow split mung dal, rinsed, soaked in water for 30 to 60 minutes, rinsed again, and drained

½ cup white basmati or baby basmati rice, washed and drained

2 tablespoons ghee or olive oil, divided

½ teaspoon ground turmeric

6 fresh curry leaves or 2 dried cassia leaves

1 tablespoon minced fresh ginger

1 small green Indian or Thai chile, seeded and minced

2 cups medium diced vegetables: carrots, zucchini, green beans, broccoli, daikon radish, asparagus, to name a few

2 teaspoons salt, or to taste

1 teaspoon ground fennel

2 handfuls chopped spinach, kale, chard, or arugula

GARNISHES

Olive oil or cultured ghee

Freshly ground black pepper

2 tablespoons chopped fresh cilantro, thyme, or basil leaves

1 slice of lime per serving

FOR VATA BALANCING: Enjoy as is.

FOR PITTA BALANCING: Replace the ghee with coconut oil, if desired. Reduce the fresh ginger to 1 teaspoon and omit the green chile. Add 1 teaspoon ground coriander with the spices in Step 2.

FOR KAPHA BALANCING: Reduce the cooking ghee to 2 teaspoons and the garnishing olive oil to 1 teaspoon. Add 1 more green chile. Substitute ¼ cup quinoa for ¼ cup of the basmati rice.

1. Heat 1 tablespoon of the ghee in a heavy 4-quart saucepan over low heat. Add the turmeric and toast for 10 seconds, then add the curry leaves, ginger, and chile and continue to toast until they crisp up, about 30 seconds. Add the lentils and rice and stir frequently until the moisture of the lentils and grains dries up, about 5 minutes. Add the vegetables, salt, ground fennel, and 4 cups water. (Add quick-cooking vegetables such as zucchini and asparagus 20 minutes into the cooking.) Bring to a full boil over medium-high heat, then lower the heat to low, cover,

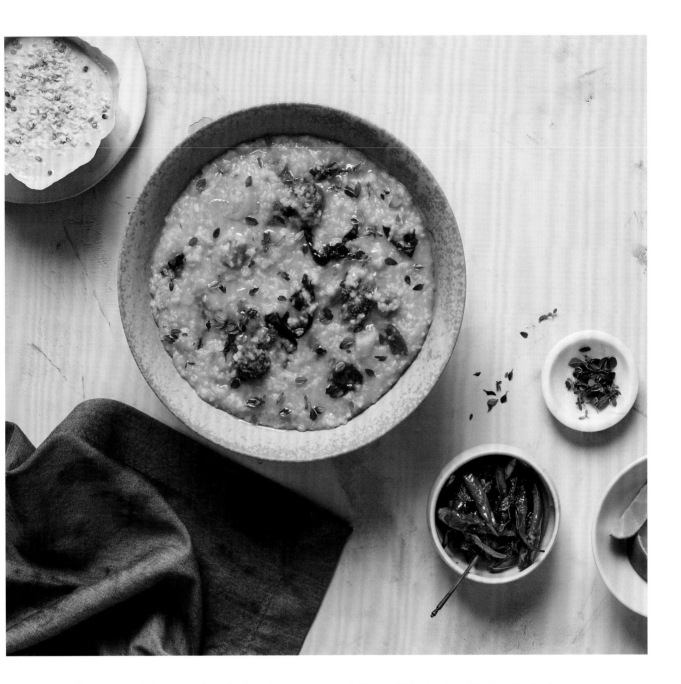

and simmer, stirring occasionally, for about 30 minutes, until the lentils begin to dissolve, the rice is soft, and the vegetables are cooked. If the kitchari dries out too much and begins to stick to the bottom of the pot, add more hot water; you're looking for a creamy, moist consistency.

2. Turn off the heat and fold in the leafy greens and the remaining 1 tablespoon ghee. Garnish each bowl with a drizzle of olive oil, a couple of turns of the peppermill, and the cilantro. Serve hot with a slice of lime on the side (to be squeezed and the juice mixed into the kitchari before eating).

Above: Simple Kitchari, Coconut Chutney, Marinated Green Chiles

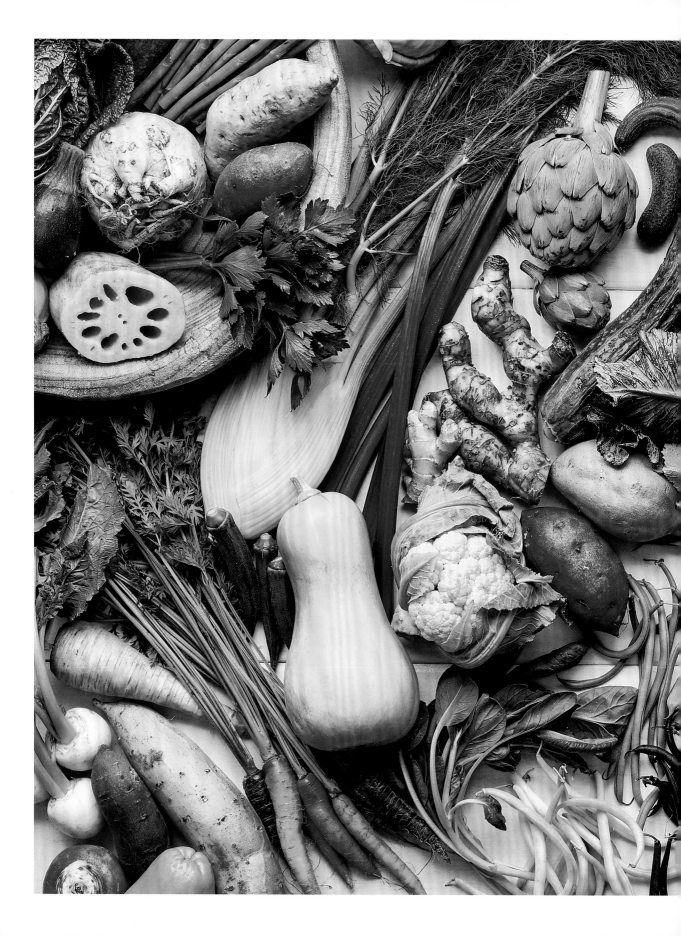

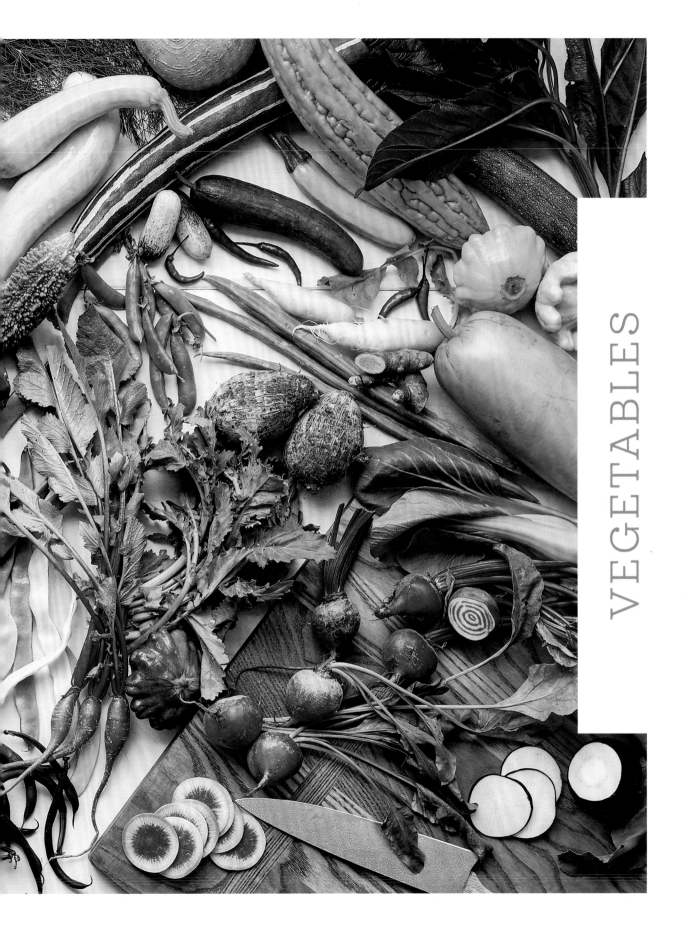

VEGETABLES

VEGETABLES

Growing up as a meat eater, I only knew a few vegetables. The basic vegetable staples in Bulgaria were potatoes, tomatoes, eggplants, peppers, spinach, squash, cabbage, carrots, beets, green beans, and cucumbers. Since becoming a vegetarian at the age of eighteen, and especially during my five-year stay in India, I discovered so many more members of the vegetable kingdom.

I could not believe the opulent produce stands at the Indian farmers markets. In any season, there were varieties of squash, various leafy greens, and exotic tubers such as taro root, ratalu, and suran. Shopping at a farmers market always deepens my appreciation for the gifts of Mother Earth.

It's interesting how the ancient Ayurveda textbooks classified vegetables, or *shaka-varga*, twenty-five hundred years ago:

- Leafy Greens
- Flowering
- Fruity
- Stems
- Tubers/Rhizomes
- Roots

The sequence of this list describes the vegetables from the easiest to the hardest to digest. Western nutrition divides vegetables as: salad, fruiting, squashes, shoots, leafy, pods, bulbs, and roots. Additional categories include cruciferous, nightshades, alliums, seaweed, and mushrooms. In *Joy of Balance*, I follow the Ayurvedic classification and outline profiles and recipes with representatives from each group.

Vegetables are indispensable to a healthy diet. They provide us with essential vitamins, minerals, and fiber that protect us from disease. I'd suggest that you research what grows in your region and when, and make it a point to rotate them on your plate throughout the year.

In the Shaka Vansiya Ayurveda tradition, we consider alliums (i.e., onions, garlic, leeks, shallots, chives) medicinal foods—we do not cook with them daily because they are quite strong and can have side effects, especially for people with Pitta disorders. In *What to Eat for How You Feel*, I explain why I choose not to include onions and garlic in my daily meals. There is nothing wrong with alliums when used occasionally as medicine.

You might notice that mushrooms are also absent in my recipes. In general, edible mushrooms are hard to digest and tend to have a clogging effect. Ayurveda considers the detoxifying properties of the numerous fungi and sets preference for white mushrooms for culinary use, but even then, still lists them as the least desirable vegetable and recommends them only for occasional consumption.

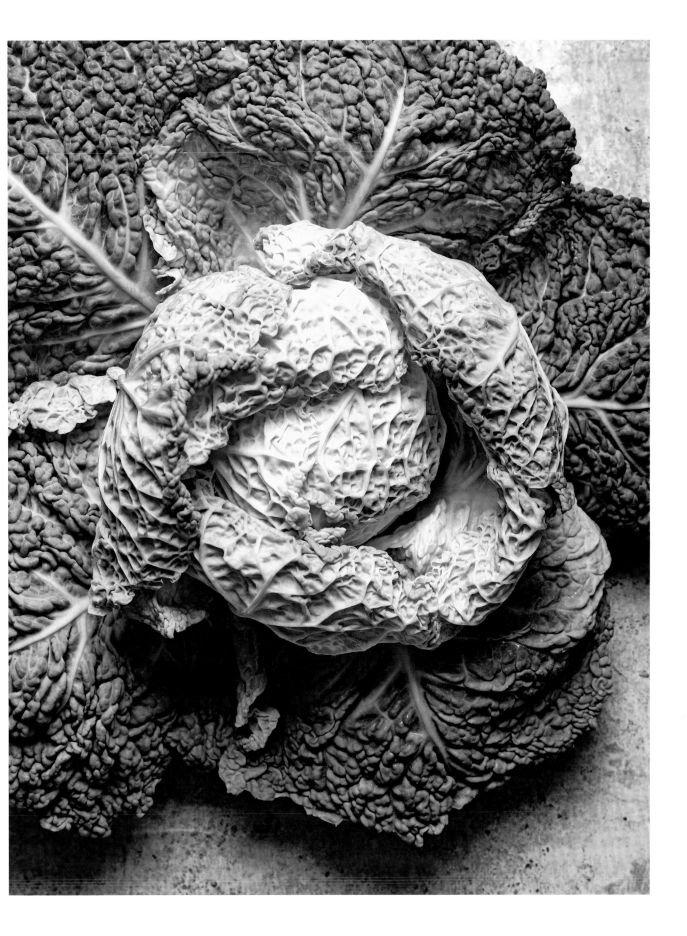

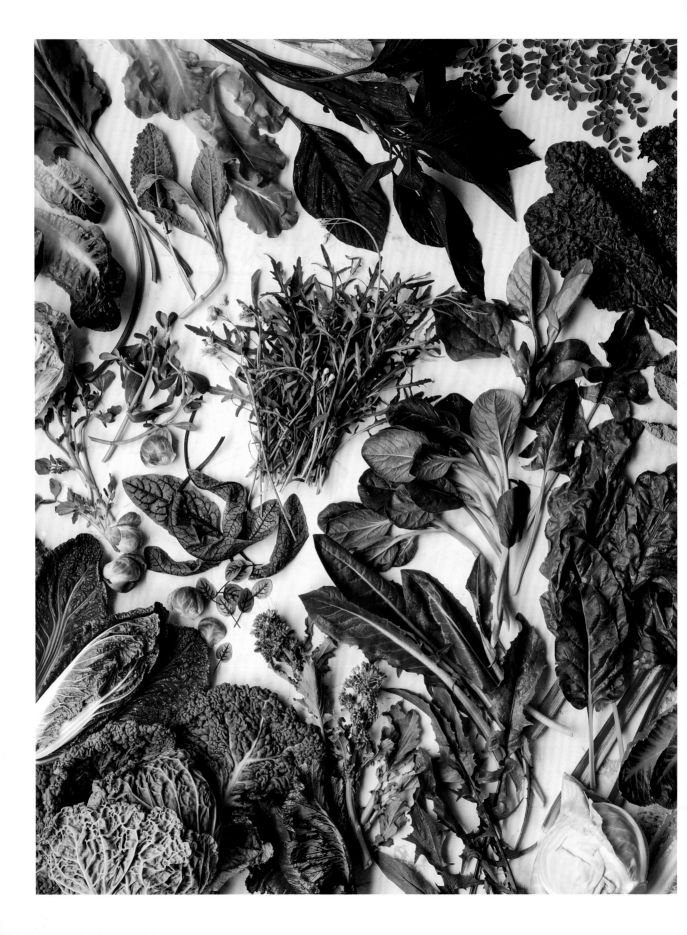

LEAFY GREEN VEGETABLES

examples:

green & purple cabbage

napa cabbage

savoy cabbage

Brussels sprouts

spinach

Malabar spinach

kale

chard

lettuces

dandelion greens

watercress

beet & radish greens

amaranth greens

broccoli rabe

arugula

sorrel

purslane

Leafy green vegetables are light to digest, being mostly of bitter or astringent tastes. Leafy greens are the foods richest in chlorophyll, which supports our blood, liver, and lungs. It is important to eat greens regularly because they replenish minerals in the body. When consumed raw (including as green juice), they will aggravate Vata. Because of their airy nature, cellulose content, and chemical composition, the best way to assimilate the nutrients from leafy greens (lettuce is an exception) is to lightly cook them in a healthy fat.

Sautéed leafy greens cook within five minutes—you want them to wilt but remain vibrant green. Gently seasoned with coriander, cumin, ginger, turmeric, or asafoetida makes leafy green vegetables suitable for everyone. I enjoy having leafy greens every day, and I rotate the different kinds for variety and nutrition.

Properly washing your leafy greens is important. The best way is to plunge the greens in a bowl of cold water; lift them up, discard the water and then wash again, until there are no dirt particles lingering at the bottom of the bowl. If you will not be using all of the washed leafy greens right away, store them in a vegetable bag in the refrigerator produce drawer, and use them soon, as they spoil fast.

broccoli rabe and beets with saffron almonds

SERVES 4 ● **PREP:** 15 minutes ● **COOK:** 15 minutes ● **GF, DF** ● **SPRING-SUMMER**

This recipe was featured in episode 6 of season 3 of the PBS show *Lucky Chow*. The host (and one of the sweetest women I've ever met), Danielle Chang, asked me to cook a recipe together with her—specifically, a recipe to promote beautiful skin.

Is there a connection between the food you eat and the glow of your skin? Yes, absolutely! Ayurveda describes skin disorders in great detail, and a lot of them start with poor digestion. You've probably noticed a pimple or skin dryness manifesting when you're constipated, when you eat certain foods, or when you're dehydrated.

This bitterly delicious and colorful dish is tridoshic. It helps flush sludge from the liver and gallbladder and supports healthy bile production, which in turn helps with optimal digestion. A healthy liver and bile sift and drive out toxins. Broccoli rabe and beets also act as blood purifiers and blood builders. Clean blood = clean skin. To add to the glow, I use saffron-infused almonds as a garnish. Saffron is the number one herb used in Ayurveda to enhance overall complexion. Cultured ghee benefits the skin by moisturizing it from within. Ghee increases *ojas* (linked to vitality)— that natural glow that no skin product can produce.

Another bonus of this recipe: it helps reduce sugar cravings!

Broccoli Rabe and Beets with Saffron Almonds goes well with Plain Basmati Rice (page 64), Millet Pilaf with Grated Carrots (page 60), Lime Rice Pilaf (page 65), Dill-Mung Soup with Vegetable Noodles (page 89), and more.

2 teaspoons coriander seeds

½ teaspoon fennel seeds

¼ teaspoon cumin seeds

4 teaspoons ghee or olive oil, divided

½ teaspoon kalonji seeds

1 teaspoon salt, divided

2 small or 1 medium red or candy cane beet, peeled and shaved thin into rounds or wedges (about 2 cups; see Notes)

1 tablespoon slivered fresh ginger

1 green Indian or Thai chile, seeded and minced

¼ teaspoon ground turmeric

1 medium bunch broccoli rabe, bottom stems discarded, upper stems thinly sliced, and leaves chopped into 1-inch strips (about 5 cups total)

¼ teaspoon freshly ground black pepper

2 teaspoons fresh lime juice

GARNISHES

⅛ teaspoon (a small pinch) saffron threads, crushed

2 tablespoons slivered almonds

CONTINUED

Opposite: Broccoli Rabe and Beets with Saffron Almonds, Marinated Paneer Cheese, Two Ways

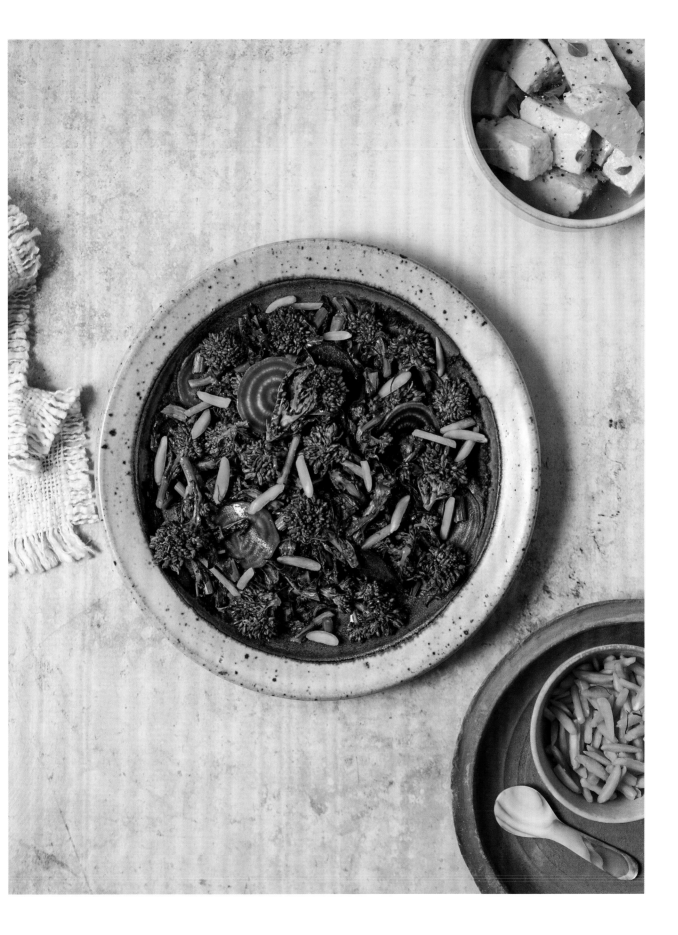

FOR VATA BALANCING: Enjoy as is.

FOR PITTA BALANCING: Omit the chile.

FOR KAPHA BALANCING: Reduce the ghee or olive oil to 2 teaspoons.

1. In an electric spice grinder, grind the coriander, fennel, and cumin seeds to a powder.

2. Heat a small skillet over medium-low heat. Add 2 teaspoons of the ghee and the kalonji seeds, and toast for about 5 seconds, until the seeds release their aroma. Then add 1 teaspoon of the ground spice blend and ¼ teaspoon of the salt. Toast for 5 more seconds, then add the beets. Mix well and sauté, stirring occasionally, for about 5 minutes, until the beets are soft. If they begin to brown and stick to the pan, splash in a little water. Transfer the cooked beets to a bowl and set aside, covered.

3. Wipe clean the same skillet (or use a different pan), and heat the remaining 2 teaspoons ghee over medium heat. Add the ginger, chile, and turmeric. Toast for about 10 seconds, until the ginger crisps up, then add the remaining ground spice blend and the remaining ¾ teaspoon salt. Fold in the broccoli rabe, cover, and cook for about 1 minute, until the greens wilt. Continue to sauté uncovered, tossing frequently until the broccoli rabe is soft yet still vibrant green, about 5 minutes.

4. Turn off the heat and sprinkle both the beets and broccoli rabe with the pepper and lime juice.

5. To make the saffron almonds garnish: In a small skillet or a metal measuring cup, heat 2 teaspoons water over medium-low heat. Add the saffron and toast for 5 seconds, or until the strands release their yellow color. Add the slivered almonds and shake and toast for a minute or so, until the water evaporates and the almonds become crisp and bright yellow.

6. To assemble it all, lay the broccoli rabe in a serving dish of your choice, top with the beets, and garnish with the saffron almonds. Or mix the broccoli rabe and beets together and garnish with the almonds. Serve immediately.

NOTE: To thinly shave the beets in an easy way, use a mandoline, a spiralizer, or the shaving side of a box grater.

CAUTION: Broccoli rabe is detoxifying—do not eat it if you're pregnant or nursing.

creamy spinach with paneer cheese

PALAK PANEER

SERVES 2 ● **PREP:** 10 minutes (with already made paneer cheese) ● **COOK:** about 10 minutes ● **GF** ●
SUMMER-FALL-WINTER

Spinach (*palak*) with fresh cheese (*paneer*) is perhaps one of the most beloved North Indian dishes, served at practically every Indian restaurant. What many people don't notice is the heavy cream that is used in a lot of the common recipes for this dish. Ayurveda warns us that milk or heavy cream are incompatible with salty or sour foods—eating such combinations can cause skin disorders. In the common recipes, the heavy cream clashes with the salt, cheese, tomatoes, and lemon. In this recipe, I replace the heavy cream with "paneer cream," which I make by blending the leftover bits and pieces of cubing the paneer with a little water. This paneer cream lends the comforting creamy consistency we all love so much, but without the side effects from the food incompatibility.

In this recipe, I also show you a different method of cooking with spices: toasting a spice paste in ghee. I use this method whenever I want the whole seeds and spices to remain "invisible."

Enjoy Creamy Spinach with Paneer Cheese in the cold season and in the summer; it might be too heavy for you in the spring. It goes well with rice, flatbreads, and dal soup.

2 teaspoons coriander seeds

¼ teaspoon cumin seeds

¼ teaspoon fenugreek seeds

¼ teaspoon ground turmeric

1 teaspoon finely grated fresh ginger

1 tablespoon ghee or olive oil

8 ounces (7½ cups) washed, stemmed, and drained fresh spinach

6 ounces pressed paneer cheese (page 205, made from 6 cups milk), cut into ¾-inch cubes (1½ cups)

1 ounce (about 2 tablespoons) paneer cheese bits and pieces (the remains of cutting the paneer block into cubes)

¾ teaspoon salt

1 teaspoon fresh lime juice

GARNISH

Freshly ground black pepper

FOR VATA OR PITTA BALANCING: Enjoy as is.

FOR KAPHA BALANCING: Add 1 seeded and minced green Indian or Thai chile with the ginger in Step 1. Reduce the ghee or olive oil to 2 teaspoons.

1. Using an electric spice grinder, grind the coriander seeds, cumin seeds, fenugreek seeds, and turmeric to a powder. Add the ginger and 2 tablespoons water, and grind briefly to turn the spices into a paste.

2. Heat the ghee in a 12-inch sauté pan over medium-low heat. Add the spice paste and toast for about 15 seconds, until it mixes well with the ghee. Fold in the spinach and gently

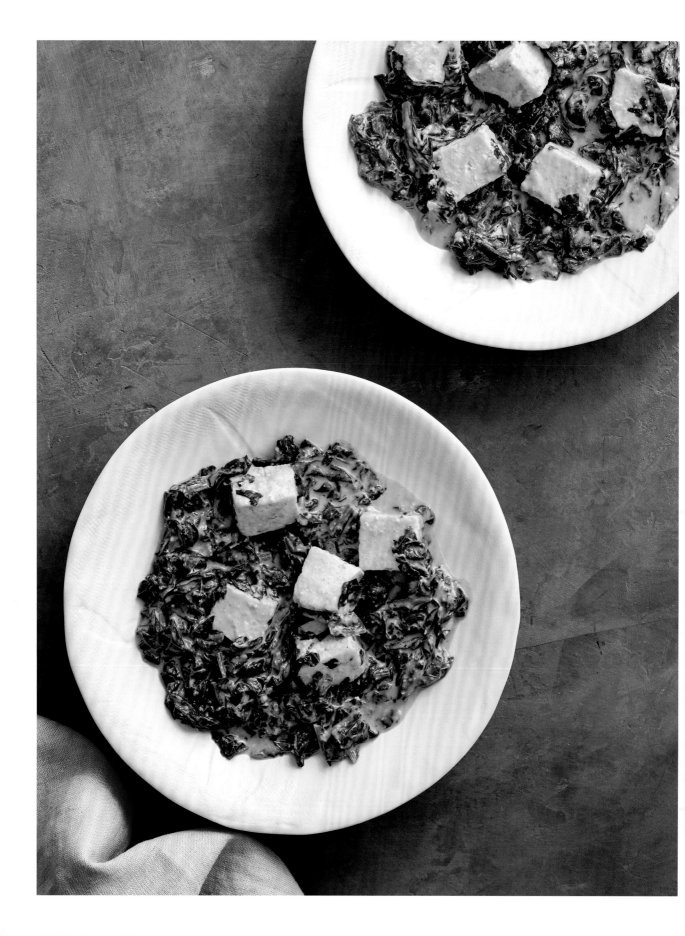

turn it around (salad tongs are very convenient for turning greens) until most of the spinach wilts yet remains vibrant green, about 3 minutes. Add the paneer cheese cubes and gently stir. If the ingredients look too dry, add about a tablespoon of water. Continue to simmer uncovered for 2 to 3 minutes; the spinach should remain vibrant green.

3. In the meantime, place the bits and pieces of cheese, the salt, and ⅓ cup water in the spice grinder (no need to wash from Step 1) or a small blender. Blend until you achieve a smooth, heavy cream–like consistency.

4. Fold the paneer cheese cream into the cooking spinach and cheese, and continue to simmer for another 5 minutes, allowing the cream to blend well with the ingredients and the cheese cubes to become very soft.

5. Turn off the heat and leave the pan uncovered for a couple of minutes. Just take a moment and let your eyes bathe in the sight of the dark leafy greens and white cheese cubes mingling in a velvety pale-yellow cream while your nose enjoys the most captivating aroma!

6. Fold in the lime juice. Serve hot, garnishing each serving with a pinch of black pepper.

VARIATION: Substitute thinly sliced beet greens, chard, kale, amaranth, or other leafy greens for the spinach.

spring greens soup

SERVES 3 to 4 ● PREP: 10 minutes ● COOK: 25 minutes ● GF, DF ● SPRING

There are different types of soup—creamy, clear, brothy, cold. Ayurveda recommends the heavier, creamy soups for late fall and winter and the lighter, brothier soups for spring or when digestion tends to get weaker. Leafy greens are essential in our diet, especially during the spring. Not only do they provide us with essential minerals and vitamins but they also aid the natural detoxification functions of our body.

This recipe is inspired by Yamuna Devi, and I really enjoy it during the spring months. I find the clear and spicy broth mixed with ribbons of bright leafy greens and specs of yellow millet to be very nourishing and invigorating. It reminds me of a baby nettles soup my father used to make. As soon as the weather warmed up and nature revived its green covers, my father wandered in the woods, picked crisp baby nettles, and made us a soup. "It will give you lots of iron," he said. I continue to follow this tradition in New York City, only that I forage my nettles from the farmers market instead of from the woods.

Spring Greens Soup pairs well with Vegan and Gluten-Free Bread (page 57), Adzuki Bean and Red Lentil Patties (page 84), or Celery Root and Taro Pancakes (page 153).

1 tablespoon + 1 teaspoon ghee or olive oil, divided

½ teaspoon black mustard seeds

2 tablespoons millet or quinoa (wash the quinoa)

2 teaspoons salt

1 or 2 green Indian or Thai chiles, seeded and minced

1 teaspoon ground coriander

¼ teaspoon ground turmeric

4 cups hot Quick Vegetable Stock (page 143) or hot water

4 cups washed and thinly sliced spring greens (chard, spinach, stinging nettles, beet greens, to name a few)

2 tablespoons fresh lime juice

GARNISH

Freshly ground black pepper

FOR PITTA BALANCING: Omit the chile and reduce the mustard seeds to ¼ teaspoon.

FOR VATA OR KAPHA BALANCING: Enjoy as is.

1. Heat 1 tablespoon of the ghee in a 3-quart saucepan over medium-low heat. Add the mustard seeds and toast them until they turn gray and start popping. Add the millet, salt, chile, coriander, and turmeric, and mix and toast them for about 30 seconds, then add the hot stock and 3 cups water and bring to a boil. Cover, lower the heat to low, and simmer for 15 to 20 minutes, until the grains are done.

2. While the grains are cooking, heat the remaining 1 teaspoon ghee in a medium skillet over medium heat. Add the greens and sauté them for 2 minutes, or until they wilt but are still vibrant green. Set aside.

3. Fold the sautéed greens and lime juice into the cooked soup. Garnish each bowl with a pinch of black pepper and serve hot.

steamed kale salad

SERVES 3 to 4 ● PREP: 20 minutes ● COOK: 1 minute ● GF, DF ● YEAR-ROUND ● Photograph on page 85

I've noticed that Ayurvedic practitioners often recommend their clients to minimize the amount of raw salads they eat because it requires strong digestion, which a lot of people lack nowadays. The alternative is a steamed salad as I show with this recipe, which will still deliver the crunch, colors, and flavors that you enjoy in the raw options.

Enjoy this Italian-style salad all year around. It pairs well with a lentil soup, quinoa, rice, bean patties, pasta, paneer cheese, and more.

1 bunch kale (about 15 leaves), washed and stems removed

1 medium carrot, peeled and cut into matchsticks (about ½ cup)

4 small red radishes or 1 small watermelon radish, peeled and sliced into wedges (about ¼ cup)

3 tablespoons dried cranberries

2 tablespoons halved pitted black olives

DRESSING

1 tablespoon fresh lime juice

1 tablespoon fresh ginger juice (see Note)

½ teaspoon dried basil

¼ teaspoon salt

¼ teaspoon freshly ground black pepper

2 tablespoons olive oil

GARNISH

2 tablespoons toasted pine nuts, slivered almonds, or walnuts

FOR PITTA BALANCING: Enjoy as is or omit the olives and black pepper if you have acidic digestion.

FOR VATA OR KAPHA BALANCING: Enjoy as is.

1. Add enough water to a medium saucepan so it comes just a couple of inches below the base of a steaming basket set atop. Bring to a boil over medium heat. Add the stripped kale leaves, cover, and steam for 1 minute. Use tongs to transfer the kale from the steamer to a large tray, spreading the leaves apart to allow them to cool. Chop the kale into bite-size pieces (whatever size is easiest for you to chew).

2. Transfer the kale to a serving bowl, then toss in the carrots, radishes, cranberries, and olives.

To make the dressing:

3. In a small bowl, whisk the lime juice, ginger juice, basil, salt, and pepper, then gradually whisk in the olive oil.

4. To toast the nuts, heat a small skillet on low and add the nuts. Move them frequently on the pan until they turn slightly golden in color. Transfer the nuts to a small bowl, and let them cool completely.

5. About 10 minutes before serving, toss in the dressing and let the salad marinate. Garnish each serving with nuts. Serve at room temperature.

NOTE: To make ginger juice, grate a 2-inch piece of ginger, wrap it in a small cheesecloth or muslin cloth, and use your hand to twist and squeeze out the juice.

green tabbouleh

SERVES 4 ● PREP: 20 minutes ● COOK: 20 minutes ● GF, DF ● YEAR-ROUND

Tabbouleh is a traditional Middle Eastern salad served as an appetizer, but I think my Ayurvedic take on it can easily become a simple meal during the spring and summer. The inspiration behind this recipe is Melina Takvorian-Mishra, the wife of my late teacher, Vaidya R. K. Mishra. I've learned so much from her about how to "Ayurvedize" recipes.

This salad is very colorful and fresh tasting. The vibrant greens fleck with red, orange, and black vegetables, and the white quinoa paints an image of a righteously healthy bowl. After eating it, you will feel that you ate something very nutritious yet so light. For variety, you could add to it more steamed vegetables such as beets and sunchokes, raw cucumbers, or jicama.

Green Tabbouleh goes well with Roasted Sweet Potatoes (page 149), Adzuki Bean and Red Lentil Patties (page 84), and Gluten-Free Paratha Flatbread (page 56). You could also pack this tabbouleh as travel food, keeping the dressing in a separate little container. It's a convenient way to eat a nutritious meal that tastes delicious at room temperature.

⅓ cup white quinoa, washed and drained

¼ teaspoon + a pinch of salt, divided

½-inch chunk fresh ginger, peeled and chopped

6 fresh curry leaves

½ green Indian or Thai chile, seeded (optional)

1 bunch kale (about ½ pound), washed, stems removed, and torn into smaller pieces

1 teaspoon olive oil

Tiny pinch of asafoetida

¼ cup finely diced (⅛-inch) carrots

2 or 3 red radishes, diced (¼-inch)

2 tablespoons finely diced (¼-inch) celery

¼ cup chopped pitted black olives

DRESSING

2½ tablespoons olive oil

2 tablespoons fresh lime juice

1 teaspoon salt (or less, depending on how salty the olives are)

¼ teaspoon freshly ground black pepper

GARNISHES

¼ cup toasted pine nuts or walnuts

2 tablespoons fresh parsley leaves

1 tablespoon fresh mint leaves

FOR PITTA BALANCING: Omit the chile.

FOR VATA OR KAPHA BALANCING: Enjoy as is.

CONTINUED

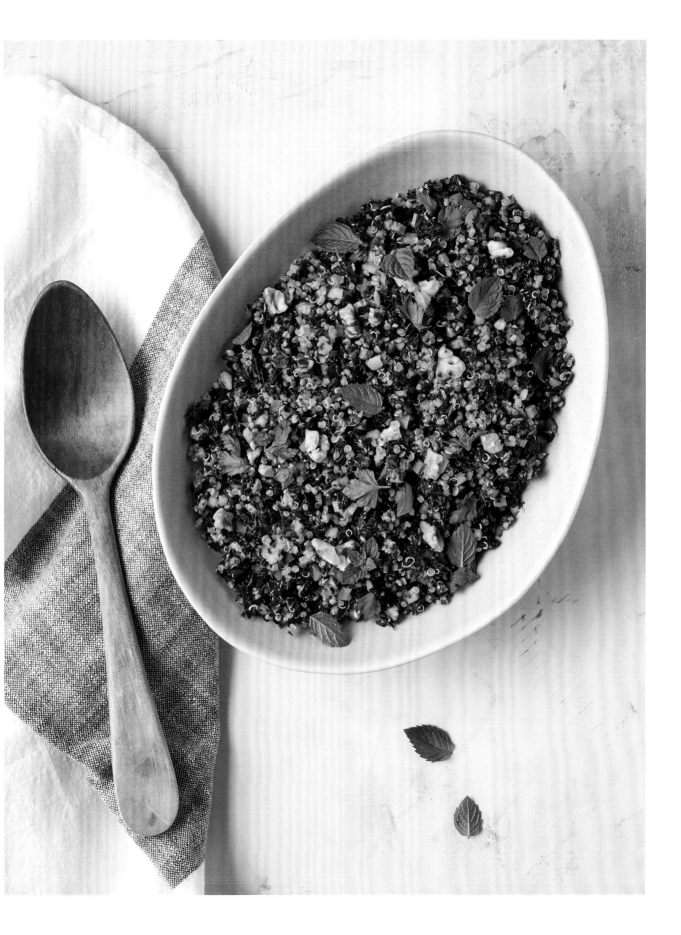

1. In a medium saucepan, bring 3 cups water to a boil over medium-high heat, then add the quinoa and ¼ teaspoon of the salt. Cook uncovered for 12 to 15 minutes, until the grains are done (a little tail-shoot will separate from the seed). Drain well. Spread on a plate or tray to let the quinoa cool completely.

2. In a food processor, finely chop the ginger, curry leaves, and chile. Add the kale leaves and pulse until they are finely chopped but not pasty. (If your food processor is small, you might need to chop the kale in two or three batches.)

3. In a 10-inch skillet, heat the olive oil over low heat. Add the asafoetida, chopped and seasoned kale, and the carrots. Sauté for about 3 minutes, until the kale wilts but is still vibrant green and the carrots are softer but still crunchy. Season with a pinch of salt and set aside to cool.

To make the dressing:

4. In a small bowl, whisk the olive oil, lime juice, salt, and black pepper.

5. To toast the pine nuts, heat a small skillet on low and add the nuts. Move them frequently on the pan until they turn slightly golden in color. Transfer the nuts to a small bowl, and let them cool completely.

To assemble:

6. In a large bowl, combine the quinoa, kale and carrots, radishes, celery, and olives. Just before serving, drizzle the dressing over the tabbouleh and toss to mix. Serve at room temperature, and garnish each bowl with pine nuts, parsley, and mint.

VARIATION: To add more protein, cook ⅓ cup French or black beluga lentils with 1 cup water and ¼ teaspoon salt in a small saucepan, uncovered, until the lentils are tender but not mushy, about 20 minutes. Drain and cool, then mix in with the salad in Step 5.

stuffed cabbage rolls

MAKES 10 rolls ● **PREP:** 40 minutes (with already made paneer cheese and cooked rice) ●
COOK: 35 minutes ● **GF, DF OPTION** ● **FALL-WINTER**

I have this vivid childhood memory from growing up in Bulgaria: stuffed cabbage rolls at every Christmas. They were the special holiday dish that gathered the whole family around the table, each one of us taking responsibility for executing a step of the recipe.

Yes, this dish is time-consuming, but it is an opportunity for a long, joyous time spent with family and friends. This is one of those dishes that requires a couple of hours to make and cook but just a couple of minutes to disappear from the table. After your first attempt, you'll see it is totally worth it!

In this recipe, I put an Ayurvedic spin on the flavors, which do not compare to the ones we used when we cooked these rolls in Bulgaria. Nevertheless, they lend a most flavorsome eating experience. The sweetness of the carrots and paneer cheese balance the astringency of the cabbage and walnuts. For an elevated sensual indulgence, I recommend eating these rolls using your hands—bite into a soft filling with an occasional carrot-walnut crunch wrapped in a delicately crisp cabbage leaf topped with a custardy gravy. Take your time with each bite, and notice the subtle nuances of flavor unfolding on your palate. Take a breath and then another bite.

Stuffed Cabbage Rolls is a festive dish for the cold season and goes well with Sweet Potato and Green Bean Salad (page 151), Pineapple-Hibiscus Drink (page 168), and more.

CABBAGE

1 small savoy or green cabbage

2 teaspoons salt

SPICE CREAM

2 tablespoons macadamia nuts or cashews

¼ teaspoon cumin seeds

¼ teaspoon black peppercorns

⅛ teaspoon ground turmeric

Tiny pinch of ground cinnamon

FILLING

1½ teaspoons ghee

1½ teaspoons olive oil

2 teaspoons peeled and finely minced fresh ginger

¼ teaspoon salt, or to taste

Tiny pinch of asafoetida

½ cup finely diced (¼-inch) carrots

2 ounces (½ cup) crumbled soft paneer cheese (page 205) or ½ cup soaked cashew pieces

½ cup walnuts, finely chopped

1 cup cooked Plain Basmati Rice (from ⅓ cup uncooked rice, page 64)

2 tablespoons minced fresh dill

1 tablespoon fresh lime juice

Olive oil

GARNISHES

1 cup Cashew Gravy (page 185)

1 tablespoon minced fresh dill

CONTINUED

FOR VATA OR PITTA BALANCING: Enjoy as is.

FOR KAPHA BALANCING: Add 1 seeded and minced green Indian or Thai chile with the ginger in Step 5, or serve the rolls with an additional hot sauce.

To blanch the cabbage leaves:

1. Cut off the core at the bottom of the cabbage head, and remove any damaged or torn outer leaves. Using a paring knife, carefully cut the leaves at their base to remove and separate the 10 most outer leaves (each one about 6 or 7 inches in diameter); make sure these leaves remain without tears.

2. Fill a 4-quart saucepan with 3 quarts water and bring to a boil; add the salt. Blanch 5 leaves at a time until the leaves are crispy tender and pliable but not soft (4 to 5 minutes for savoy cabbage, or 5 to 6 minutes for green cabbage). Gently transfer the leaves to a colander, and rinse them with cold water. Line them on kitchen towels or paper towels to absorb excess water. Repeat with the remaining 5 leaves.

3. Working with one leaf at a time, position the leaf in a convex way (dome-shape), so the thick part of the leaf's spine faces up. Keeping the leaf intact, use a paring knife to carefully trim the thick, protruding part of the outer leaf spine that runs from the middle to the base of the leaf. You want the base of the leaf to be thin and pliable enough to roll. Set aside and repeat with the remaining leaves.

To make the spice cream:

4. In an electric spice grinder or a small blender, grind the macadamia nuts, cumin seeds, peppercorns, turmeric, and cinnamon to a powder. Add ½ cup water and briefly blend to create a thin paste.

To make the filling:

5. Heat a 10-inch skillet over medium-low heat. Add the ghee and olive oil and then the ginger, salt, and asafoetida. Toast for 5 to 10 seconds, until the ginger crisps up, then add the spice cream; mix well. Add the carrots, paneer cheese, and walnuts. Sauté for up to 5 minutes, until the carrots are softer yet still crunchy. Fold in the cooked rice and turn off the heat. Add the dill and lime juice and mix well. Adjust the salt to your liking. (If not stuffing the leaves immediately, refrigerate the filling until you're ready to use it.)

6. Preheat the oven to 400°F. In a 9 x 9-inch baking or casserole dish, pour in just enough water to cover the bottom.

To stuff the cabbage leaves:

7. Spread one leaf on a flat surface in a concave position (bowl-shape; inner side of the leaf facing up and the cut base closest to you), and place about 2 tablespoons of the filling in the center of the leaf (the amount of filling will vary according to the size of the leaf). Fold the left and right sides over the filling, then the side closest to you. Next, tightly roll it toward the last unrolled side (away from you). This technique is similar to rolling sushi or a burrito. Place the roll in the prepared baking dish, seam-side down. Repeat with the remaining leaves.

8. Lightly drizzle olive oil over the rolls and bake for 15 to 20 minutes, until they form a light golden crust.

9. As soon as you take the rolls out of the oven, artistically pour some of the Cashew Gravy on top of them. Garnish with the dill. Serve hot, with extra gravy on the side.

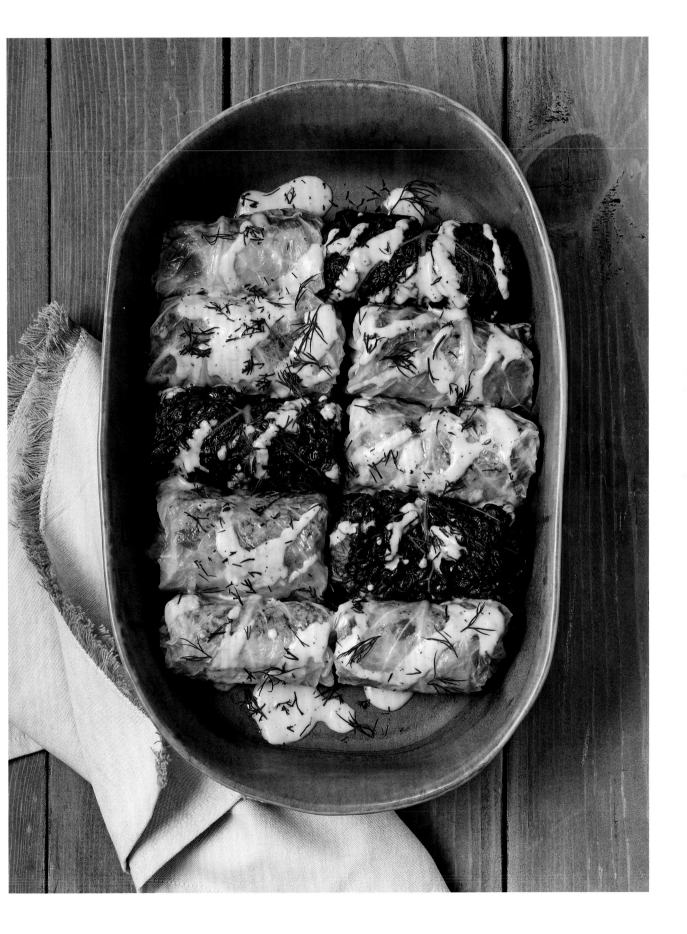

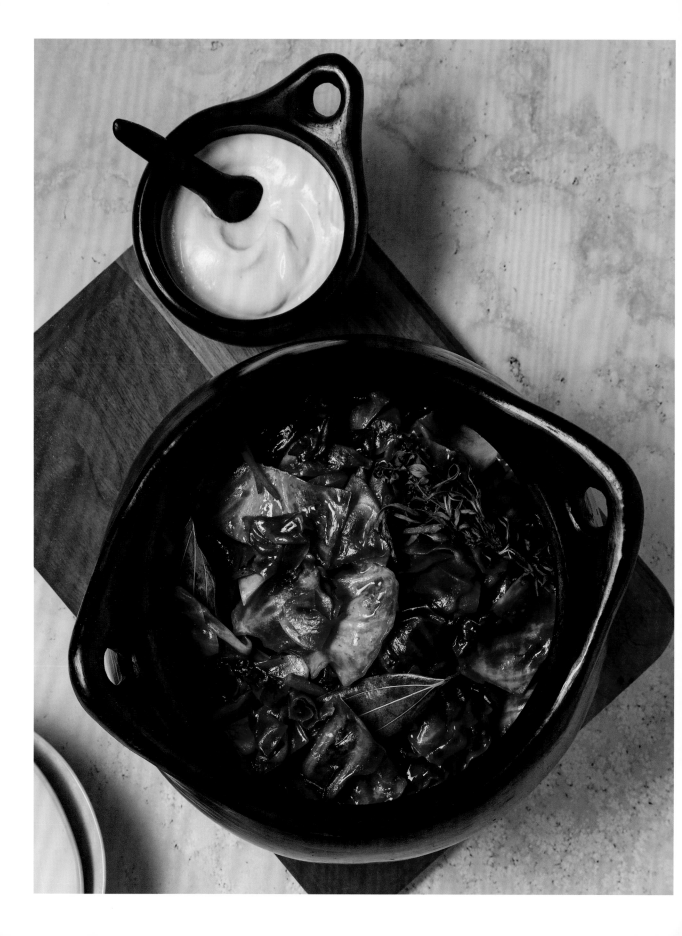

braised purple cabbage

SERVES 2 to 3 ● PREP: 10 minutes ● COOK: 45 minutes ● GF, DF ● WINTER-SPRING

This cabbage dish is so simple yet so attractive with its regal purple color and deeply comforting texture. I love braising cabbage because it adds sweetness to its astringent, sulphury taste, and it creates a mouth-melting eating experience. Cabbage in general is Vata aggravating, but I find the braising method to make it and other cruciferous vegetables Vata friendly. If you're not crazy about cabbage, this recipe might change your feelings.

Braised Purple Cabbage is most balancing in the late winter and spring. It goes well with Marinated Paneer Cheese, Two Ways (page 206), Sautéed Mung Sprouts (page 92), Millet Pilaf with Grated Carrots (page 60), Plain Basmati Rice (page 64), Lime Rice Pilaf (page 65), Cashew Sour Cream (page 186), Roasted Carrot Tahini Sauce (page 148), and more. Try to eat it all as soon as you cook it because the color and flavor of this dish become less pleasant within an hour after cooking.

2 tablespoons ghee or olive oil

2 teaspoons thinly julienned fresh ginger, 1 inch long

4 whole cloves

2 bay leaves

1 teaspoon salt

1 teaspoon ground fennel

¼ teaspoon freshly ground black pepper

Tiny pinch of asafoetida

1 small head purple cabbage (about 1½ pounds), cored and cut into 2-inch pieces

2 cups Quick Vegetable Broth (page 143) or water

2 sprigs fresh thyme

1 sprig fresh tarragon

GARNISH

2 teaspoons fresh lime juice

FOR VATA BALANCING: Enjoy as is.

FOR PITTA BALANCING: Omit the asafoetida and reduce the ginger to 1 teaspoon.

FOR KAPHA BALANCING: Enjoy as is or add 1 seeded and minced green Indian or Thai chile with the ginger in Step 2.

1. Preheat the oven to 350°F.

2. Heat the ghee in a medium-large clay pot, Dutch oven, or other ovenproof pot over low heat. Add the ginger and toast for 10 seconds, then add the cloves, bay leaves, salt, fennel, pepper, asafoetida, and cabbage. Increase the heat to medium-high and sauté for 3 to 4 minutes, until the cabbage combines well with the spices. Pour enough hot broth to cover the vegetables by about one-third, and add the thyme and tarragon sprigs. Bring to a simmer, then turn off the heat.

3. Cover the cabbage with a piece of parchment paper cut to the inner diameter of the pot, then cover the pot with a tight-fitting lid, and transfer to the oven.

4. Braise in the oven for about 40 minutes, until the cabbage is very tender. Remove and discard the parchment paper, herb sprigs, and bay leaves. Garnish with the lime juice and serve hot.

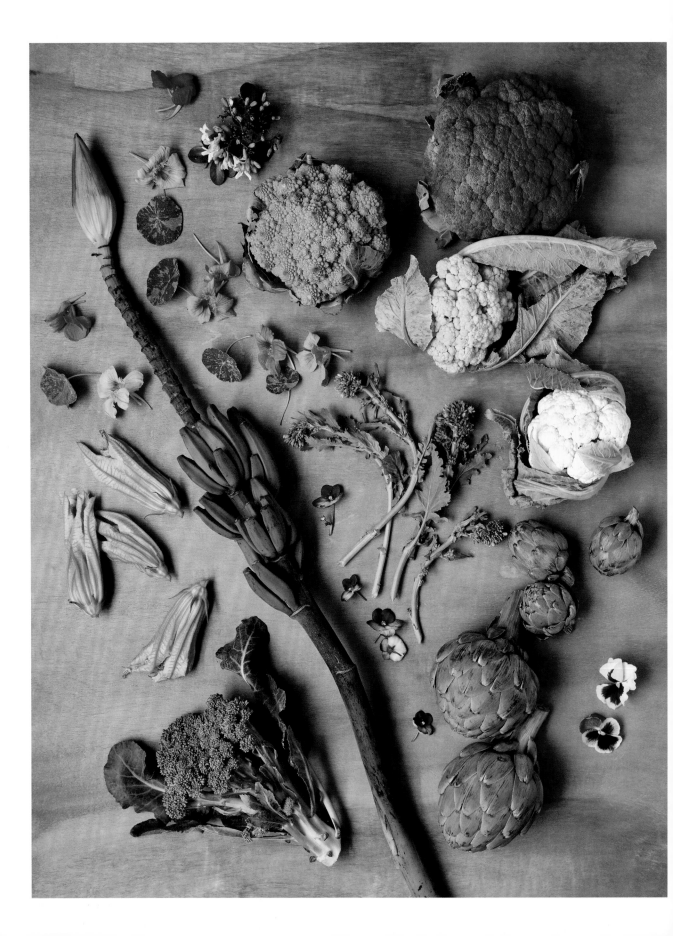

FLOWERING VEGETABLES

examples:

zucchini blossoms

banana flowers

artichoke

cauliflower

broccoli

nasturtiums

rapini flowers

borage

Like leafy greens, flowering vegetables are easy to digest and of airy nature. With the exception of edible flowers for decoration, these vegetables need to be cooked to assure proper absorption by the body.

Make sure to use the stems of cauliflower, broccoli, or artichokes, as they are more nutritious than the actual crowns. These vegetables are a good source of potassium, calcium, and vitamins A and C.

cauliflower soup with almond cream

SERVES 4 to 6 ● SOAK: 8 hours or overnight ● PREP: 20 minutes ● COOK: 20 minutes ● GF, DF ●
FALL-WINTER-SPRING

As a cruciferous vegetable, cauliflower is excellent for balancing the Kapha and Pitta doshas, but it may aggravate the Vata dosha. Even if you are one of those people who have scratched cauliflower from their shopping list, try this soup. It should cause you no airy problems because it is balanced with fresh almond cream and spices. It is the kind of velvety, comforting, delicious treat you need on a brisk winter day.

I served this soup at the Autism Speaks Celebrity Chef Gala at Cipriani on Wall Street in October 2017. Guessing by the empty bowls and happy faces, I think the ten guests at our table loved this dish.

Cauliflower Soup with Almond Cream goes well with Plain Basmati Rice (page 64), Gluten-Free Paratha Flatbread (page 56), Red Rice with Spinach and Nuts (page 63), and more.

2 tablespoons ghee, sesame oil, or
   coconut oil

½ teaspoon ground turmeric

½ teaspoon cumin seeds

6 fresh curry leaves

2½ teaspoons salt

Tiny pinch of asafoetida

1 small cauliflower, cut into 2-inch florets;
   stems and smaller greens chopped
   (6 cups total)

2 medium taro roots, peeled and sliced
   ¼ inch thick (about 1 cup)

½ cup almonds, soaked in water for at least
   8 hours or overnight, drained, and rinsed

¼ teaspoon freshly ground white pepper,
   or to taste

GARNISH

2 tablespoons parsley leaves or minced
   fresh dill

1. Heat the ghee in a 4-quart saucepan over medium-low heat. Add the turmeric and toast for 10 seconds, then add the cumin seeds and toast for 5 more seconds. Add the curry leaves, salt, and asafoetida, and toast for about 10 more seconds, until the leaves crisp up. Add the cauliflower and taro, stir to mix the vegetables with the spices, and sauté for 2 to 3 minutes. Add 5 cups water, increase the heat to medium-high, and bring to a full boil. Cover, lower the heat, and simmer until the cauliflower and taro are tender, about 15 minutes.

2. Meanwhile, prepare the almond cream: To peel off the skins of the soaked almonds easily, cover them with a cup of boiling hot water for a few seconds. Rinse, drain, and peel the almonds. In a blender, blend them with ⅔ cup water to a smooth cream. Set aside ¼ cup of the cream for garnishing.

3. Let the cooked soup sit uncovered for 10 minutes to cool down a bit, then add the pepper and blend the soup with the almond cream to your preferred consistency: chunky or smooth (add more water if necessary). I prefer it smooth, so once it's blended, it looks like delicate custard.

4. Reheat the soup. Garnish each bowl with the fresh herb and a swirl of almond cream. Serve immediately.

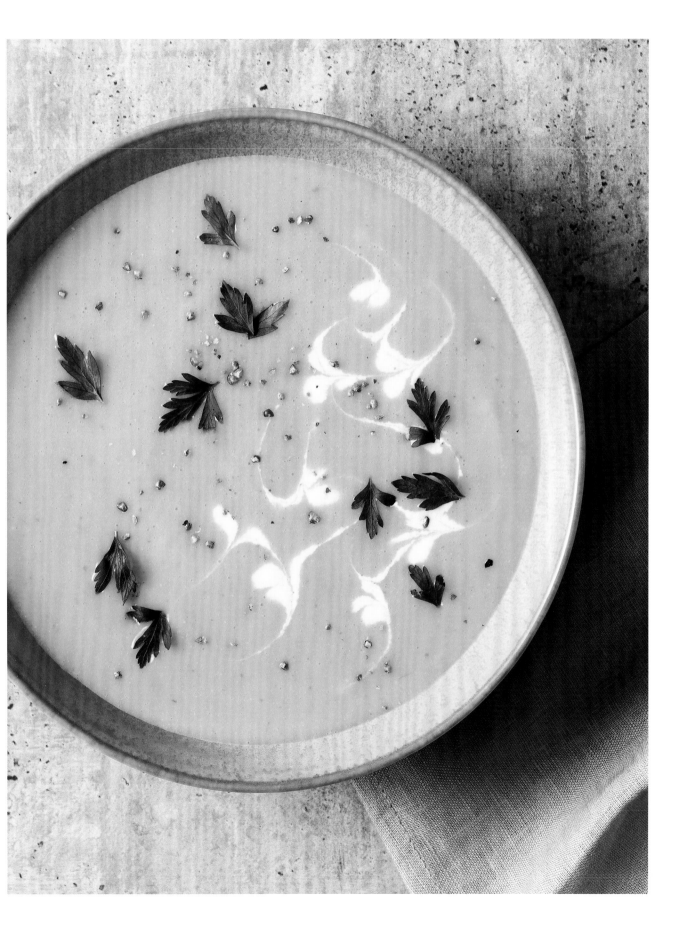

STALK AND STEM VEGETABLES

examples:

asparagus

celery

rhubarb

bamboo shoots

kohlrabi

fennel stalks

bok choy stems

chives

scallions

cardoons

broccoli stems

lotus stems

fiddleheads

chard stems

Stalks and stems are of less variety but equal importance. Not all stalks and stems of plants are edible, but the ones I list and discuss here are. From a culinary perspective, they can be just as much a part of the plant as are its roots, leaves, and seeds. Just like the stem of a plant transports nutrients from its roots to its crown, branches, and leaves, the human body utilizes stem vegetables in a similar fashion—they move energy and matter, specifically the stagnant kind, out and away.

You've probably noticed that ridged stems tend to have quite stiff fibers—think of the rough "threads" woven in a celery or fennel stalk. When you eat these fibers and you feel like they cause bloating, then this means they're too rough for your gut, and it is best to shave them off with a peeler.

Choose firm and vibrant stem vegetables, and keep them wrapped in a damp cloth or plastic bag in the refrigerator to preserve their crispness. When you buy a fennel bulb or a head of broccoli, don't discard the stems—use them! I like to stir-fry, roast, sauté, or steam them as a part of my meal, or I simmer them in a vegetable broth.

ASPARAGUS

"Asparagus Pee Is Real, but Only Some of Us Can Smell It"—this was the headline of a *HuffPost* article that grabbed my attention. If you've noticed that your pee smells funky after eating asparagus, there is nothing to worry about—this happens to everyone, but some can't smell it. And just in case you're wondering, the smell generates after our body breaks down the asparagusic acid that's abundant in the stalk. This is no reason to stop eating this delicious and very nutritious vegetable.

In the kitchen, we use garden asparagus, which is not to be mistaken with *Asparagus racemosus*, commonly known as the herb shatavari. Asparagus is my go-to vegetable when I need to fix a quick meal—it requires very little effort to prepare, and it cooks in five minutes.

BOTANICAL NAME ● *Asparagus officinalis*

SANSKRIT NAME ● not available

AYURVEDIC ATTRIBUTES

TASTE ● astringent, sweet

QUALITIES ● light to digest, bulky

METABOLIC EFFECT ● cooling

POST-DIGESTIVE EFFECT ● sweet

DOSHA EFFECTS ● balances all three doshas

HEALING BENEFITS ● acts as a diuretic, is rich in antioxidants, energizes the kidneys, lungs, and spleen

SOURCING

● You can find asparagus at the farmers market and grocery stores. The stalks vary in thickness. They spoil quickly, so examine the spears carefully to ensure vibrant green crisp tips. If the tips are mushy and smell bad, the asparagus is past its prime. Refrigerate the stalks upright in a container with water (like a bouquet in a vase). Among the green, purple, and white varieties, I prefer the green because it is richer in chlorophyll.

SEASON

● Asparagus grows for a short period during the spring. If my kidneys need help, I would also eat it out of season because of its ability to cleanse them.

DIGESTIBILITY

● Asparagus is easy to digest and is one of the few vegetables that are good for everyone. I like to add ground coriander to an asparagus dish to further support its diuretic and detoxifying properties. You will pee more, but since bad stuff is going out, you shouldn't mind this so much.

COOKING TIPS

● The bottom ends of the spears are woody and fibrous, making them hard to chew and digest. Cut off these parts: an easy way to determine where this line is, is to hold a spear on each end and bend it until it snaps. Keep the longer, softer side and discard the other piece, or use it for broth.

● Take advantage of the many ways to cook asparagus: steam, sauté, roast, or boil it.

● For kidney support, cook asparagus with daikon radish and ground coriander.

EAT ASPARAGUS WHEN YOU NEED TO

● reduce inflammation,

● clean your kidneys,

● eliminate kidney stones,

● lower cholesterol,

● induce a delayed menstrual period,

● increase breast milk supply, and/or

● counteract the side effects, of radiation and chemotherapy.

CAUTION ● Avoid asparagus when you're pregnant or following a low-estrogen diet.

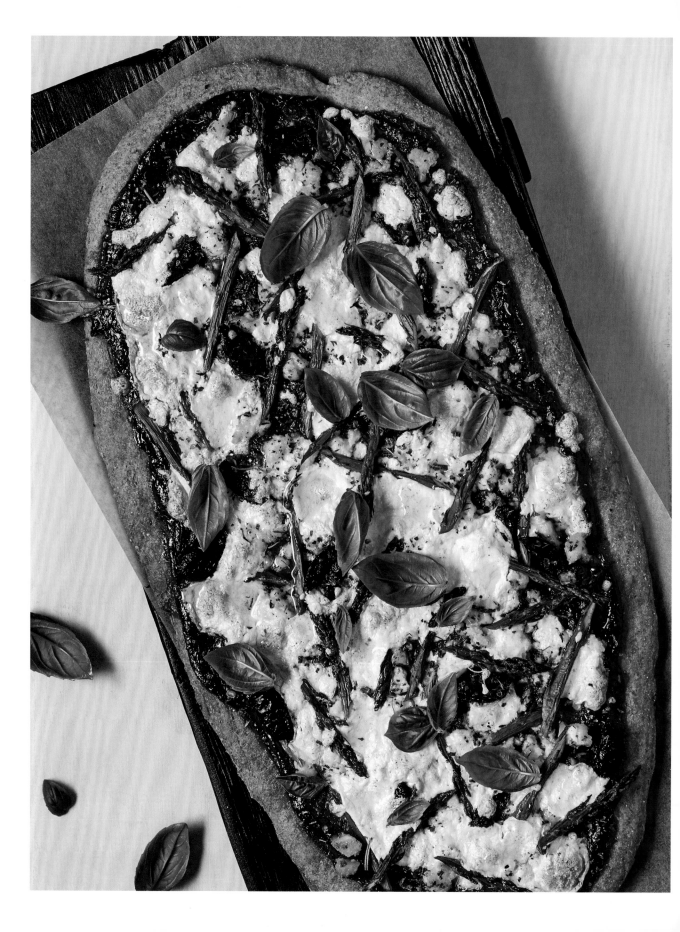

asparagus pizza

MAKES 1 medium pie ● **PREP:** 25 minutes (with already made paneer cheese and "Ketchup") ● **BAKE:** 15 to 20 minutes ● **SPRING-SUMMER**

I like my pizza full of flavor, with a thin and crispy crust and a generous topping. This makes me feel that I'm eating a meal of substance, not just low-nutrient comfort food. For a few years, I avoided pizza because of the yeast in the crust (the yeast really disturbs Vata in the gut). One year, my husband, Prentiss, expressed an undeniable birthday wish: pizza! I created two recipes for him—this one and a pie with white sauce, spinach, and paneer cheese. He loved them both.

The crust for this pizza is quick to make because you don't have to wait for the dough to rise. It is yeast-free, so it resembles more of a tart dough, not the common pillowy pizza dough. You can keep the dough wrapped and refrigerated for 4 to 6 hours, and take it out to room temperature 30 minutes before you're ready to roll it. You can also use this dough to make breadsticks or a tart base.

The toppings take a little work, but you can prepare them ahead of time, and you can switch them up. With all the prep done in advance, assembling and baking this pie is fairly quick and easy.

With its vibrant Italian flag colors—green, white, and red—and its fresh, nutrient-dense ingredients, Asparagus Pizza is a delicious, less inflammatory version of the traditional recipe. My hard-core Italian foodie friends vouch for it, and that is good enough for me.

CRUST

1¾ cups (205 grams) whole spelt flour

1 teaspoon baking powder

¼ + ⅛ teaspoon salt

¼ cup olive oil

⅓ cup + 2 tablespoons buttermilk

1 teaspoon fresh lime juice

TOPPING

2 tablespoons olive oil

Tiny pinch of asafoetida

⅓ cup Ayurvedic "Ketchup" (page 173), divided

8 stalks asparagus, trimmed, cut into 2-inch-long pieces, and halved lengthwise (no need to half if the asparagus is pencil-thin)

4 ounces (¼ cup) crumbled soft paneer cheese (page 205)

¼ teaspoon salt

¼ teaspoon freshly ground black pepper

1 teaspoon Italian seasoning

1 tablespoon sliced olives

1 tablespoon torn fresh basil leaves

¼ cup grated fresh mozzarella cheese

½ teaspoon dried oregano

GARNISHES

Olive oil

A few fresh basil leaves

CONTINUED

To make the crust:

1. Mix the flour, baking powder, and salt in a large bowl.

2. Rub the oil into the flour mixture with your fingertips until it resembles a coarse meal. Add the buttermilk and lime juice, and briefly work it to a soft but not sticky dough. (If it's too sticky, add a little more flour.) Do not knead the dough too much, just enough to mold all ingredients into a ball. Wrap the dough with a damp kitchen towel or plastic wrap and refrigerate for 10 minutes.

3. Preheat the oven to 400°F. Have a half-size sheet pan or a pizza stone ready.

4. Lightly dust a silicone mat or a piece of parchment paper (taping it on the counter-top can make it easier to roll) and a rolling pin with flour, press the dough into a smooth disk, and then roll it into your desired shape (round or oblong), ¼ inch thick. Transfer to the sheet pan.

To make the topping:

5. Whisk the olive oil and asafoetida in a small bowl or cup. Brush the rolled dough with half of the asafoetida-infused olive oil and with a very thin layer (about 2 tablespoons) of the Ayurvedic "Ketchup."

6. Partially bake for about 7 minutes, until it forms a soft crust.

7. Spread the remaining "ketchup" on the crust. Then arrange the following ingredients in this order: asparagus, soft paneer cheese, salt, pepper, Italian seasoning, olives, basil, mozzarella, oregano, and the remaining asafoetida-infused olive oil.

8. Bake until the top has patches of golden-crusted ingredients, about 10 minutes.

9. Slice and serve hot, garnished with olive oil and basil leaves.

VARIATION: Substitute 1 or 2 steamed and sliced artichoke hearts for the asparagus.

FRUITING VEGETABLES

examples:

zucchini

lauki squash

ash gourd

snake gourd

butternut squash

pumpkin

green beans

fennel bulb

peas

chayote

bitter melon

okra

tomato

eggplant

peppers

cucumber

avocado

A plant can have several edible parts, each falling into a different group of vegetables. For example, we cook with zucchini blossoms and zucchini fruit, radish root and radish leafy greens, and fennel bulb, stalks, and greens. In our daily cooking, we might not speak of "fruiting" or "fruit" vegetables, but this is the technical name of a vegetable that is the fruit of a plant.

Among the fruiting vegetables, Ayurveda considers the white-fleshed summer squashes to be the best. Ash gourd and lauki squash (a.k.a. bottle gourd) are listed among the most healing types because they are a good source of Soma energy: nurturing, hydrating, and cooling for the liver. They thrive in warmer climates and are frequently sold at Indian or Asian grocery stores. In the West, it is easier to access yellow and pattypan squash, zucchini, and Lebanese zucchini, all of which have similar properties to the traditional Ayurvedic gourds.

Vegetables of the nightshade family—tomatoes, potatoes, eggplants, and peppers—are sources of some good nutrients, but they are difficult to digest and can increase or perpetuate inflammation. I grew up eating them with practically every meal, so my body is accustomed to them. However, I significantly reduced my nightshade consumption when I had an autoimmune disorder. Now I enjoy them occasionally when they are in season, and especially when I have the luxury of picking them from my mom's garden.

summer curry

AVIAL

SERVES 3 to 4 ● PREP: 15 minutes ● COOK: 30 minutes ● GF, DF OPTION ● SUMMER

This Summer Curry delivers the flavors of South India, but its fame descends from the ancient Puranic texts and narratives of the warrior Bhima and his brothers. You can prepare *avial* anywhere in the world, using regional produce.

The concept of *avial* is cooking whatever local vegetables you have available and combining them with a yogurt-coconut sauce. The dish has a succulent and semidry consistency (dryer than other curries), and it glows bright yellow. It feels very refreshing to eat this dish during the hot summer.

My recipe calls for five specific vegetables, but you can replace some of them with other local produce of different colors: parsnips, baby turnips, flat beans, sweet potato, moringa pods (drumsticks), snake gourd, broccoli, cauliflower, and more. Avoid leafy greens, as they are incompatible with dairy yogurt (nondairy yogurt is okay).

Summer Curry is a plentiful vegetable dish that goes well with plain rice, flatbreads, lentils, bean patties, salad, and more. If you choose to eat this curry for two meals, keep the second portion of vegetables and yogurt sauce separately; reheat the vegetables, then add the sauce. Ayurveda warns us against reheating yogurt.

1 tablespoon coconut oil or ghee

5 fresh curry leaves

1 green Indian or Thai chile, seeded and minced

½ teaspoon ground turmeric

1¼ teaspoons salt, divided

1½ cups peeled and cut (¾-inch) lauki squash or zucchini (no need to peel zucchini)

1 small fennel bulb, chopped into ¾-inch pieces (about 1 cup)

1 small taro root, peeled and cut into ¾-inch pieces (about ⅔ cup)

1 medium carrot, peeled and sliced ¼ inch thick (about ⅔ cup)

½ cup trimmed and cut (1 inch long) green beans

½ cup plain whole yogurt or nondairy yogurt

⅓ cup fresh or dried shredded coconut

GARNISH

2 tablespoons fresh cilantro leaves

1. Heat the coconut oil in a 12-inch skillet over medium-low heat. Add the curry leaves, chile, turmeric, and 1 teaspoon salt and toast for 10 seconds. Add the squash, fennel, taro, carrots, and green beans. Sauté, stirring frequently, for 5 minutes (if using zucchini, add it 15 minutes into the cooking). Add ½ cup water and bring to a simmer. Lower the heat to low, cover, and simmer, stirring occasionally, for 20 to 30 minutes, until the vegetables are tender and have absorbed most of the liquid.

2. In a small bowl, whisk together the yogurt, coconut, and the remaining ¼ teaspoon salt. Gently fold the mixture into the cooked vegetables. Cover and set aside for 5 minutes to incorporate the flavors.

3. Garnish with cilantro and serve immediately.

Opposite: Summer Curry (Avial), Gluten-Free Paratha Flatbread, Aloe Vera Mint Cooler

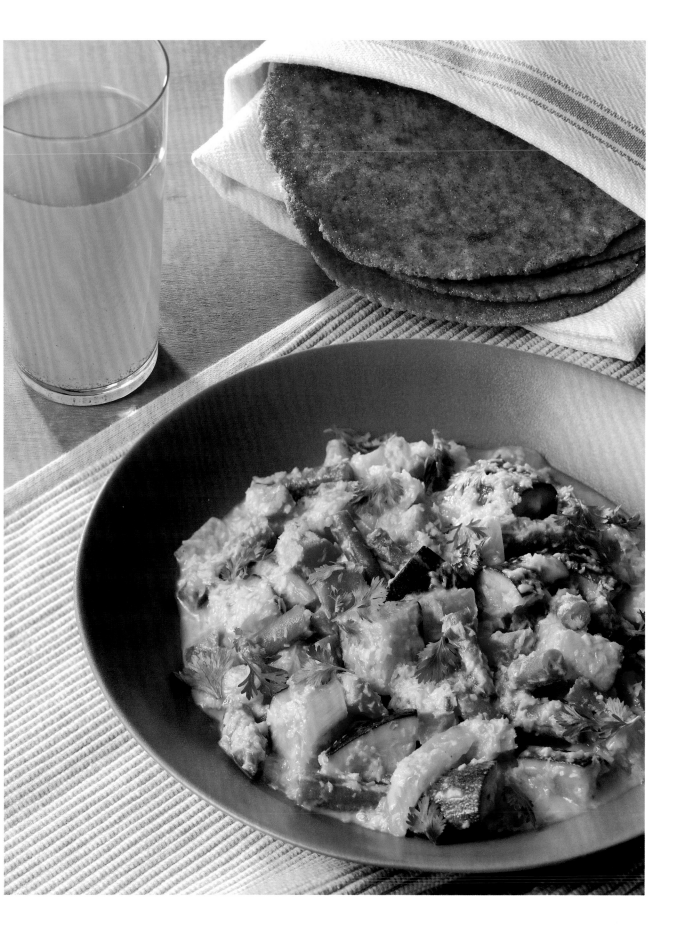

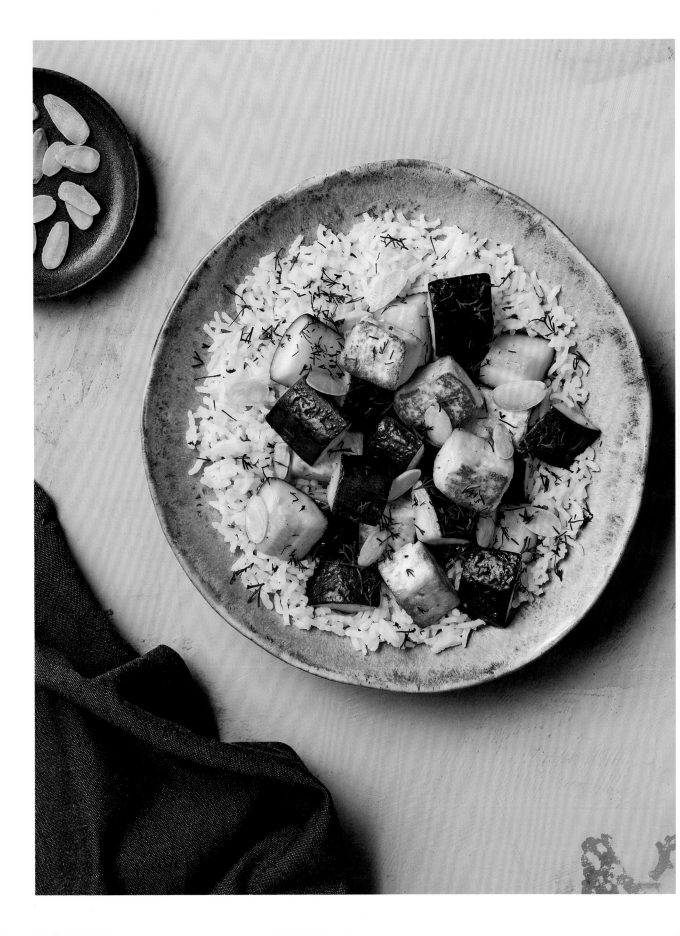

zucchini with paneer cheese and toasted almonds

SERVES 4 • **PREP:** 10 minutes (with already made paneer cheese) • **COOK:** 15 minutes • **GF** • **SUMMER**

Vaidya Mishra recommended zucchini to most of his patients. This easy-to-digest summer vegetable draws heat out of the liver and thus helps cool down the whole body. I also love it because it is easy to find and so versatile for cooking.

This stir-fried dish pleases with simple flavors and quick preparation—perfect for a hot summer day when you don't feel like doing much cooking. Serve it with Plain Basmati Rice (page 64) and a salad with Sunflower-Herb Dressing (page 193).

3 tablespoons sliced almonds or whole pine nuts

1½ tablespoons ghee or olive oil, divided

¾ teaspoon salt, divided

¼ teaspoon freshly ground black pepper

⅛ teaspoon asafoetida

2 medium zucchinis (about 1 pound), trimmed and chopped into ¾-inch cubes (3 cups)

1 tablespoon grated fresh ginger

6 ounces pressed paneer cheese (page 205, made from 6 cups milk), cut into ¾-inch pieces (1½ cups)

GARNISHES

1 tablespoon minced fresh dill

1½ teaspoons fresh lime juice

FOR VATA BALANCING: Enjoy as is.

FOR PITTA BALANCING: Enjoy as is, or if you feel overheated, omit the black pepper and asafoetida.

FOR KAPHA BALANCING: Add 1 minced and seeded green Indian or Thai chile with the cheese in Step 3.

1. Heat a wok or skillet over medium-low heat. Add the almonds and toast them until they turn tan in color. Transfer them to a small bowl and reserve for garnishing.

2. Wipe the wok, and heat ½ tablespoon of the ghee over medium-low heat. Add ¼ teaspoon of the salt, the pepper, asafoetida, and zucchini. Increase the heat to medium-high, and stir-fry by frequently moving the vegetable pieces with a metal spatula until they soften but are still crunchy and some develop a golden crust, about 5 minutes. Add the ginger, and continue to stir-fry for another minute. Transfer to a serving dish and cover.

3. Add the remaining 1 tablespoon ghee and the remaining ½ teaspoon salt to the wok, and heat over medium heat. Add the cheese cubes, and gently stir-fry them, tossing frequently, to give them a light golden crust, about 5 minutes. Turn off the heat.

4. Gently combine the stir-fried zucchini and cheese. Garnish with the dill, lime juice, and toasted almonds. Serve immediately.

cooling lauki squash

SERVES 3 or 4 ● PREP: 5 minutes ● COOK: about 15 minutes ● GF, DF ● SUMMER

Once, at the end of summer, I experienced an immense heat in my body—it rose to my head and made me feel dizzy. Soon I was hyperventilating. My symptoms escalated to the point of needing to go to the emergency room, where I was hooked up to an IV. All of my test results came back normal, and the doctors could not figure out what was causing my symptoms. Although I received excellent care at the hospital, I felt unsettled because my suffering was real, scary, and unresolved.

When I got home, I called Vaidya Mishra. He asked me detailed questions and determined that I had an episode of a severe high Pitta spike. (The potential cause was a few of my poor choices over the past couple of days: spending too much time in the hot sun without covering my head and without eating my meals on time.) Vaidya then taught me this recipe as the safest and most therapeutic food for someone who feels overheated or struggles with hyperacidity in their stomach. I ate it for three days and felt significant improvement after just the first day. I'm sharing this story so that you can learn from my mistakes: don't skip or delay a meal, don't spend too much time outdoors during the peak hot hours (especially without wearing a hat), and always stay hydrated.

If you can't find lauki, use yellow squash or zucchini for this recipe. Cooling Lauki Squash goes well with Plain Basmati Rice (page 64), Coconut Chutney (page 177), Gluten-Free Paratha Flatbread (page, 56), and more.

1 pound lauki squash, peeled and cut into ½-inch pieces

1 teaspoon ghee or coconut oil

½ teaspoon Soma Salt, or to taste

2 green cardamom pods, slightly crushed open on one end

¼ teaspoon ground turmeric

OPTIONAL GARNISHES

Splash of fresh lime juice

Fresh cilantro or mint leaves

1. In a medium sauté pan, bring ⅓ cup water to a boil over medium-high heat, and add the lauki, ghee, salt, cardamom, and turmeric. Cover, lower the heat to low, and simmer for about 15 minutes, until the squash is tender, plump, and translucent.

2. Garnish with a little lime juice and cilantro, if you like. Serve hot.

BITTER MELON

I can't quite remember when I first tasted bitter melon (it's not a part of Bulgarian cuisine), but I clearly recall eating it regularly when I lived in India. My main incentive to eat so much of it back then was to make my blood bitter so that the mosquitoes wouldn't bite me. I'm not sure if I successfully repelled the blood-thirsty insects, but in my attempt to do so, I fell in love with bitter melon. It lifts mental fog almost instantly!

Over the many years of teaching people how to cook this vegetable, I've seen different reactions—some people enjoy it and others detest it. There are also those who are so motivated by its superstar medicinal benefits that they are willing to give it a try despite its not-so-popular reputation. In whatever category you find yourself, I highly recommend you revisit your relationship with bitter melon.

Bitter melon was first described by Ayurveda thousands of years ago, and modern scientific research confirms the ancient findings and gives us even more reasons to make bitter melon a part of our diet. A study by Memorial Sloan Kettering Cancer Center states,

"Several active substances in bitter melon have been studied in both animals and humans. They act in the same way as insulin, by increasing the entry of glucose into cells and promoting its processing and storage in the liver, muscle, and fat. Bitter melon also prevents the conversion of stored nutrients to glucose and the release of this glucose into the blood. However, researchers have not established the dosage for lowering high blood glucose levels in diabetes. Therefore, it cannot be recommended as a replacement therapy for insulin or hypoglycemic drugs."

Hopefully such recommendations will emerge soon. This is just one of many scientific findings on bitter melon. Laboratory studies continue to explore the efficacy of the gourd in killing certain cancer cells and viruses.

It is important to include bitter melon in our diets because of its high nutritional values and powerful detoxifying properties. From a nutritional point of view, bitter melon is

- one of the best-known sources of thiamine, folate, and riboflavin,

- high in phosphorus, manganese, magnesium, and zinc,

- high in vitamins B_1, B_2, B_3, and C, and

- a good source of calcium, iron, and beta-carotene.

BOTANICAL NAME • *Momordica charantia*

SANSKRIT NAME • *Karavella*

AYURVEDIC ATTRIBUTES

TASTE • bitter

QUALITIES • light, drying

METABOLIC EFFECT • cooling

POST-DIGESTIVE EFFECT • pungent

DOSHA EFFECTS • balances all doshas, but could slightly increase Vata

HEALING BENEFITS • supports the functions of blood plasma and lymph; enhances wound healing; regulates blood issues, related liver disorders, dermatoses, high blood sugar, and bleeding; improves blood circulation; cures fever; helps with anemia

SOURCING

- There are several varieties of bitter melon throughout the world, but the two popular ones are the Indian and the Chinese. The Indian bitter melon is smaller, darker green, and has a deeply ridged skin. The Chinese variety is larger, lighter green, and has a slightly ridged skin; it's also less bitter than its Indian cousin. Vaidya Mishra told me that he preferred the Indian kind because it is more bitter and medicinal.

- Bitter melon is available from farmers markets and Asian grocery stores. Select vibrant and crisp bitter melons of dark green color, and beware of dark spots or mold. If the pith around the seeds has turned orange, the bitter melon is overripe and not ideal for use. Fresh bitter melon spoils fast; keep it refrigerated in a perforated plastic bag, and use it quickly.

SEASON

- This wrinkly green vegetable grows in the summer on elevated vines, just like the cucumber. It's also easy to grow in a large planter—I tried it one year on our rooftop garden, and it worked! Spring and summer are the best seasons to eat bitter melon.

DIGESTIBILITY

- Bitter melon is light and easy to digest. Use it as a medicinal, cleansing food for occasional consumption (up to three times per week) and not daily, unless supervised by an Ayurvedic doctor. Consuming cooked bitter melon excessively and/or eating it raw (including juiced) may lead to severe digestive problems. In the case of bitter melon overdose, eat some hot basmati rice mixed with ghee.

COOKING TIPS

- You can cook bitter melon like any summer squash: sautéed, roasted, steamed, braised, or stuffed.

- I like serving it as a side dish rather than adding it to a main dish, which would make the meal predominantly bitter.

- To balance the bitterness, cook bitter melon together with a sweet vegetable, such as taro root, sweet potato, parsnip, beet, or carrot.

- Add sour and pungent tastes (e.g., from lime juice and chile) to reduce the perception of bitterness.

- Add ground coriander when cooking bitter melon to support the timely elimination of toxins from the liver and blood.

EAT BITTER MELON WHEN YOU NEED TO

- detox (include it in your cleansing meals),
- lower blood sugar and hypertension,
- increase appetite and enhance digestion,
- thin your bile and help it flow better,
- reduce inflammation,
- expel parasitic worms,
- stimulate or increase menstrual flow,
- lose weight,
- lower cholesterol,
- overcome sugar cravings, and/or
- lower insulin intake

CAUTION: AVOID CONSUMING BITTER MELON IF YOU'RE

- pregnant or breastfeeding,
- experiencing low blood sugar, and/or
- taking diabetic or other medications (consult with your doctor first).

TOPICAL USE

Bitter melon has pain-relieving and wound-healing properties. The topical application of fresh bitter melon juice is useful to

- relieve burning sensations, dermatoses, and hemorrhoids, and/or
- alleviate joint pain.

sautéed bitter melon

SERVES 2 to 4 ● PREP: 5 minutes ● COOK: 15 minutes ● GF, DF ● SPRING-SUMMER

Think of this recipe as simple medicine for the liver and pancreas—that may not sound tasty initially, but the bitter flavor and the succulent and slightly crunchy textures come together quite pleasantly. Nowadays, our livers are so challenged because of increased stress, pollution, weakened digestion, and staying up late at night, not to mention alcohol and drug consumption. The liver is the main cleansing mechanism in our body, and Shaka Vansiya Ayurveda pays a lot of attention to keeping it "cool" and "clean." When the liver is happy, our blood, skin, eyes, gallbladder, kidneys, and emotions perform at their best.

I remember the first time I tasted bitter melon in India—its bitterness gave me a bit of a shock and took charge of the taste sensation in my mouth—I did not expect that a vegetable could be that bitter! This is why I learned to mix it with rice, chapati, or other sweet foods. It's the bitter-sweet principle at play with food. Now I really enjoy eating bitter melon; I love the light and clean feelings it gives me. And if it makes my liver better, bitter melon is king!

Treat Sautéed Bitter Melon as a tridoshic starter dish, not the main portion of your meal, as too much bitterness might imbalance your Vata or your blood sugar. It goes well with Simple Kitchari (page 94), Plain Basmati Rice (page 64), Millet Pilaf with Grated Carrots (page 60), Roasted Carrot Tahini Sauce (page 148), and more.

2 to 3 Indian bitter melons (about ½ pound), washed and patted-dried

1 tablespoon ghee or olive oil

1 tablespoon ground coriander

¼ teaspoon Protein Digestive Masala (page 233)

¼ teaspoon salt

⅛ teaspoon freshly ground black pepper

2 teaspoons fresh lime juice

1. Cut off the ends of the bitter melon, and cut it in half lengthwise. Scoop out the seeds with a small spoon; discard. Slice each piece of bitter melon across into ⅛-inch-thick pieces (you should end up with about 2 cups).

2. Heat the ghee in a medium skillet over medium-low heat. Add the coriander, masala, salt, and pepper. Toast for 5 seconds, then fold in the bitter melon, and make sure that all pieces are coated with the spiced ghee. Sauté for 5 minutes, then cover, adjust the heat to the lowest, and let the vegetables sweat for about 10 minutes, until they are tender. Splash in a little water if they start to crust onto the bottom of the pan.

3. Turn off the heat and let the cooked bitter melon rest uncovered for a minute, then mix in the lime juice. Serve hot.

VARIATION : For a roasted version of this dish (which will better balance the Kapha dosha), prepare the bitter melon as outlined in Step 1, then mix the remaining ingredients except the lime juice in a large bowl. Spread the bitter melon on a medium baking sheet, and roast at 400°F for about 15 minutes, until the bitter melon is tender, with a slight golden crust. Garnish with lime juice.

stuffed bitter melon

SERVES 4 to 5 ● SOAK: 8 hours or overnight ● PREP: 20 minutes ● COOK: 15 minutes ● GF, DF ●
SPRING-SUMMER

When it comes to cooking, which type of person are you? Do you prefer to spend less time in the kitchen and make simple, unassuming-looking food, or do you welcome the extra work for the sake of more impressive results and superior enjoyment? I'm asking you because you will have to decide with this recipe: make the less involved, baked variation, or spend a little more time slicing and panfrying to stir a culinary curiosity. I'd go with the latter version, especially when I want to make a delicious first impression of bitter melon.

I created this recipe for my spiritual mentor, Krishna Kshetra Swami (a.k.a. Dr. Kenneth Valpey). He loves bitter melon, so I wanted to make yet another preparation with it. He noted that it was kind of a "gourmet" take on bitter melon. The panfried stuffed and sliced bitter melon pieces look like sun art on your plate. Bitter is the main taste of this dish, but once it passes, pungent, sweet, salty, and slightly sour continue to entertain your taste buds.

Serve Stuffed Bitter Melon as a side dish with Ayurvedic "Ketchup" (page 173), Green Tahini Sauce (page 219), or a cilantro chutney.

5 medium bitter melons, washed

1½ teaspoons salt, divided

1 cup cashews or 1½ cups sunflower seeds, soaked in water for at least 8 hours or overnight, rinsed, and drained

1 teaspoon ground coriander

½ small green Indian or Thai chile, seeded

⅛ teaspoon ground turmeric

1 tablespoon chopped fresh parsley leaves

1 tablespoon chopped fresh basil leaves

1 tablespoon sattu flour, chickpea flour, or nutritional yeast

2 teaspoons fresh lime juice

1 tablespoon ghee or coconut oil

FOR VATA BALANCING: Enjoy as is.

FOR PITTA BALANCING: Omit the chile.

FOR KAPHA BALANCING: Enjoy as is, or use a full green chile instead of a half.

1. Trim the ends of each bitter melon, and cut them in half, across. Using a small, narrow spoon, scoop out the seeds and pith from each bitter melon half to create 10 cone-shaped pieces.

2. Bring 6 cups water to a boil in a 4-quart saucepan over medium-high heat. Add 1 teaspoon of the salt. Add the bitter melon and blanch for 5 minutes. While the bitter melon is cooking, prepare a bowl with ice-cold water. Plunge the blanched melons into the ice-cold bath, then drain them well, open-side down.

CONTINUED

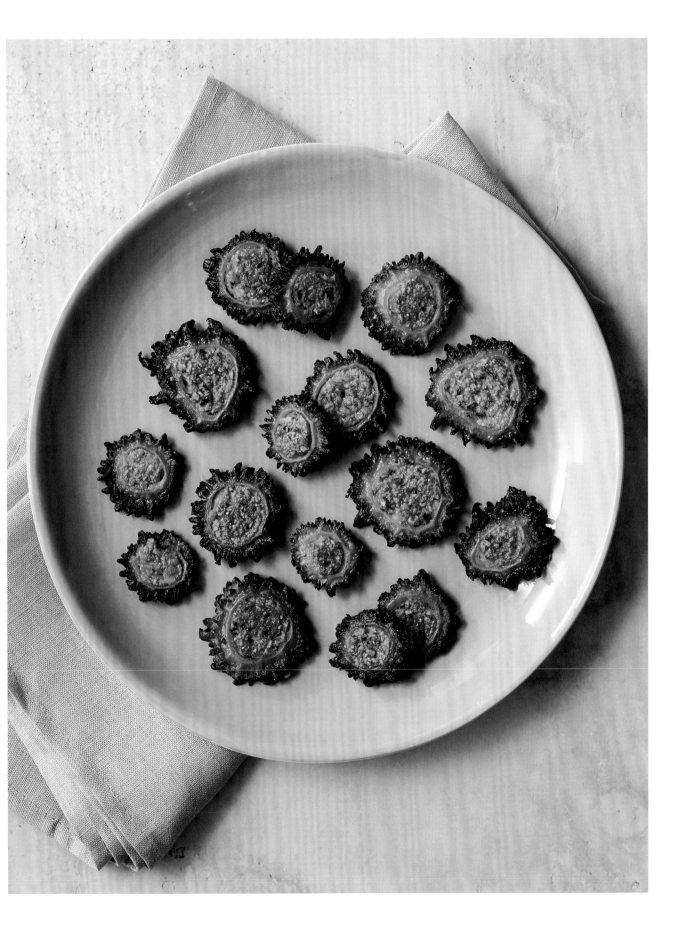

3. To make the filling, combine the cashews, coriander, chile, turmeric, and the remaining ½ teaspoon salt in a food processor, and grind to a fine meal (not pasty). Add the parsley, basil, and flour, and pulse a few times, until the herbs are chopped into small flakes.

4. Transfer the filling to a small bowl. Fold in the lime juice and ¼ cup water. The filling will have a medium-thick (not runny), sticky texture.

5. Stuff each bitter melon cone tightly with the filling. I use my index finger to push the filling all the way into the narrowest part of the cone. If you have any filling left, shape it into a patty.

6. Slice the stuffed bitter melon cones into ¼-inch-thick circles. Heat the ghee on a cast-iron griddle over medium-low heat, and add the stuffed vegetable (and plain patty if you have remaining filling). Panfry for 4 to 5 minutes on each side, until a light golden crust forms. Serve hot with your sauce of choice.

VARIATION: I find a baked version equally delicious, but less fatty and less appealing to the eye.

After Step 5, preheat the oven to 350°F. Grease a 9 x 9-inch baking pan with ghee or olive oil.

Brush the surface of each stuffed bitter melon with a thin layer of ghee or coconut oil and line the pieces onto the baking tray. Bake for about 35 minutes, occasionally rotating the pieces to make sure that they evenly bake. They will be soft and have a dull green color with a light crust. "They look ominous!" my mother-in-law, Julia, noted when she first tried the baked version. Serve hot, with your sauce of choice.

OKRA

Okra is one of those healing hero vegetables that you either love or hate. I've loved okra since I was a child. I remember my parents preserving jars of okra in tomato sauce for the winter. However, I have friends who were so put off by its slimy texture (due to improper cooking), that they signed okra off their meals for good not knowing that it is that mucilaginous gel that carries the most desirable healing benefits of this vegetable. The good news is, you can cook this vegetable without making it slimy (see Cooking Tips below).

BOTANICAL NAME • *Abelmoschus esculentus*

SANSKRIT NAME • unknown

AYURVEDIC ATTRIBUTES

TASTES • sweet, astringent

QUALITIES • dry, rough (pod), slippery

METABOLIC EFFECT • cooling

POST-DIGESTIVE EFFECT • sweet

DOSHA EFFECTS • balances Pitta and Vata, could be a little heavy for Kapha

HEALING BENEFITS • binds toxins in the blood and muscle tissues and in the liver, and then helps eliminate these toxins through the colon; lubricates the colon and eases bowel movements; decreases heat and acidity generated from toxic buildup; serves as a prebiotic; increases stamina, increases the quantity and quality of the reproductive fluid; high in carotene, B-complex vitamins, and vitamin C

SOURCING

- Buy okra from farmers markets, Indian groceries, or stores where you can hand select the pods. Packaged okra is often too old and tasteless. Choose thinner and shorter pods (under 2½ inches long), as the big pods are too fibrous and impossible to digest. Refrigerate and use the okra as soon as possible.

SEASON

- In the northern hemisphere, okra is in season during the mid-late summer.

DIGESTIBILITY

- When cooked properly (soft and vibrant but not crunchy), okra is easy to digest for all body types.

COOKING TIPS

Okra becomes slippery when it touches water—this is also called roping. The slippery sensation is due to a gooey substance called *mucilage*, which flows in the plant's leaves and also surrounds the seeds in its pod. To avoid activating the mucilage, you can try the following techniques:

- Dry the washed okra with a towel. (Or you may also wash it ahead of cooking and allow it to fully air dry by spreading it on a tray lined with a towel.)
- Make sure your hands are dry, and cut the okra with a dry knife on a dry cutting board. Dry, dry, dry.
- If you're using the whole okra pods, carefully trim off the stems, leaving the pod whole.
- Roast the whole pods at 375°F with a little ghee, salt, and ground spices such as coriander and cumin.
- If you use okra in a kitchari or a soup, sauté the whole pods separately and then add it to the dish just before serving.
- Add finely shredded coconut or a little rice flour toward the end of cooking to absorb any excess mucilage from the okra.
- Cook the okra in tomato sauce—I don't use this method, but the acidity of the tomatoes cuts the mucilage.
- Add salt at the end of cooking.

EAT OKRA WHEN YOU NEED TO

- restore or support the friendly bacteria in your gut,
- detoxify,
- heal constipation, and/or
- alleviate joint inflammation.

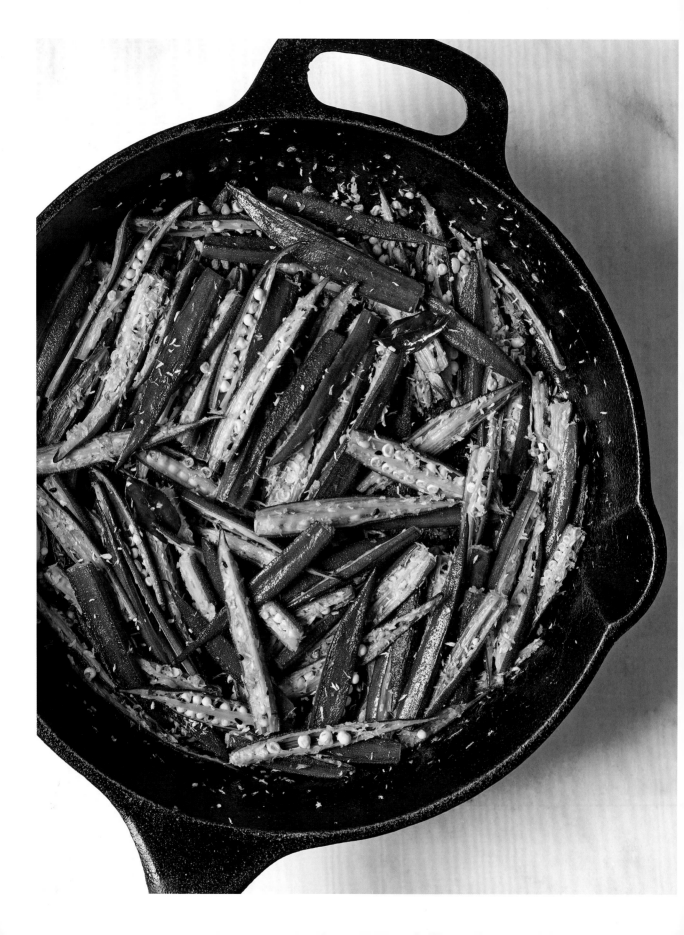

okra with coconut

SERVES 2 or 3 ● PREP: 10 minutes ● COOK: 20 minutes ● GF, DF ● SUMMER

No matter what you've thought about okra before, you've got to try this recipe. It is so tasty, it will surprise even those hesitant to experiment. Plus, okra is far too beneficial for our health to miss. Vaidya R. K. Mishra highly recommended regularly eating okra when it's in season during the summer. Eating okra while summer transitions into fall will help your body release accumulated heat so that you can enjoy the beautiful fall season without getting congested.

The trick is to cook okra properly—it should be soft and vibrant green but not crunchy; otherwise it will increase Kapha and cause indigestion.

Whenever I visit Indian grocery stores, I always notice a couple of ladies around the okra basket, grabbing and snapping off the pods' pointed ends, as if they've entered the "snatch the best okra" competition. As annoying as this ritual can be, snapping the ends is how you test the freshness of okra. (The ends of old pods will only bend, not snap.)

For a simple meal, serve this flavorful vegetable dish with Lime Rice Pilaf (page 65) or Plain Basmati Rice (page 64), Coconut Chutney (page 177), or with flatbreads.

2 tablespoons ghee or coconut oil

¼ teaspoon ground turmeric

½ teaspoon kalonji or cumin seeds

1 tablespoon minced fresh ginger

5 fresh curry leaves

¾ teaspoon ground coriander

1½ pounds okra, halved or quartered lengthwise (about 3 cups)

3 tablespoons finely grated coconut, dried or fresh

½ teaspoon salt

GARNISH

2 teaspoons fresh lime juice

FOR VATA OR PITTA BALANCING: Enjoy as is.

FOR KAPHA BALANCING: Add 1 seeded and minced green Indian or Thai chile with the ginger in Step 1.

1. Heat the ghee in a large skillet over low heat. Add the turmeric and toast for 10 seconds, then add the kalonji seeds and toast for another 10 seconds, or until the spices release their aroma. Add the ginger, curry leaves, and coriander, and continue to toast and crisp them for another 10 seconds; add the okra. Toss well, increase the heat to medium-low, and sauté, shaking or stirring frequently but gently with a metal spoon, for 10 to 15 minutes, until the okra is tender yet still vibrant green. (Be careful not to mash the vegetables while stirring.) You may cover the skillet to speed up the cooking, but do so only briefly because the condensation will make your okra slippery, giving it the dreaded "slimy" feel. If the okra begins to brown and stick to the pan, lower the heat.

2. Fold in the coconut and salt, and continue to toss and cook for 5 more minutes, or until the okra is tender and the coconut has browned slightly and absorbed the excess moisture. The vegetables will be soft and succulent, neither dry nor wet.

3. Garnish each serving with a splash of lime juice. Serve immediately.

FENNEL

Fennel is one of my favorite vegetables not only because of its versatility of cooking and flavor but also because of the soothing and calming feelings I get after I eat it.

BOTANICAL NAME ● *Foeniculum vulgare Gaertn.*
SANSKRIT NAME ● *Shatapushpa*

AYURVEDIC ATTRIBUTES

TASTE ● sweet, slightly pungent

QUALITIES ● light, oily, slightly heating

METABOLIC EFFECT ● cooling (in small amounts), heating (in large amounts)

POST-DIGESTIVE EFFECT ● sweet

DOSHA EFFECTS ● tridoshic, relieves excess Vata and Pitta in the GI tract, removes excess Kapha in the form of bronchial congestion, in large amounts the seeds aggravate Pitta

HEALING BENEFITS ● tonifies the brain, eyes, bladder, kidneys, heart, liver, and spleen; soothes the stomach by relieving flatulence, bloating, and abdominal discomfort; helps to kindle digestive fire without aggravating Pitta; acts as a mild diuretic and removes semi-digested food residue from the body; increases breast milk and stimulates the menstrual period; nourishes the plasma, blood, muscle, nerve and bone marrow

SOURCING

● Every part of the fennel plant can be used in cooking: the bulb, stalks, umbrella-like flowers, and seeds. Select small- to medium-size, unblemished bulbs that feel crisp and firm. (Some grocery stores label fennel bulbs as "anise," but the anise plant is a different species.) Look for fennel seeds that are of vibrant green color.

SEASON

● Fennel is good to eat all year round. The peak season for the fennel bulb in subtropical areas is the fall through the spring. In colder climates, it thrives in the summer.

DIGESTIBILITY

● Fennel in every form is easy to break down and enhances digestion. As a vegetable, you can use fennel as frequently as you want, and especially when you need to settle a bloated stomach or reduce congestion. Cooked fennel is easier on the intestines, but if you have a strong appetite, you could add some shaved raw bulb to a salad. I add fennel seeds as a cooling agent to balance pungent spices such as green chiles, turmeric, and ajwain.

COOKING TIPS

● Add shaved raw or steamed fennel to a summer salad.

● Braise whole fennel bulbs in the oven.

● Add the chopped bulb to vegetable or lentil soups, stir-fries, and sautéed leafy greens.

● Sauté chopped fennel with a tiny pinch of asafoetida to resemble the texture and flavor of cooked or caramelized onions.

● Add fennel seeds to breads.

● Chew (and swallow) ½ teaspoon toasted fennel seeds after meals to serve as a digestive aid.

EAT FENNEL WHEN YOU NEED TO

● counteract acidity or heartburn,

● reduce lung congestion,

● eliminate bloating or gas,

● soothe or cool your stomach, GI tract, or mind,

● increase breast milk,

● alleviate morning sickness, and/or

● increase a scant menstrual flow.

CAUTION ● Fennel in any form is a high estrogen food—avoid it when you need to lower your estrogen levels or if you're pregnant.

quick vegetable broth

MAKES 4 cups ● **PREP:** 5 minutes ● **COOK:** 10 minutes ● **GF, DF** ● **YEAR-ROUND**

Here is a quick and flavorful broth that you can use as a base for a soup or a risotto or sip on its own. Since there is no fat added, you can make this broth ahead and refrigerate it for up to two days.

½ cup sliced fennel stalks or celery

3 sprigs fresh parsley or 1½ teaspoons dried parsley

8 fresh mint leaves, chopped, or ¾ teaspoon dried mint

1 teaspoon coriander seeds

¾ teaspoon Warming Masala (page 233)

½ teaspoon salt

½ teaspoon black peppercorns

In a 2-quart saucepan, bring 4 cups water to a boil over medium-high heat and add all the ingredients. Cover, lower the heat, and simmer for 10 minutes. Strain and discard the cooked ingredients; use the broth as directed in a recipe, such as Dill-Mung Soup with Vegetable Noodles (page 89).

cream of fennel soup

SERVES 4 ● **PREP:** 15 minutes ● **COOK:** 25 minutes ● **GF, DF** ● **YEAR-ROUND**

With its smooth and delicate texture and sweet, licorice-like flavor, this soup delivers a bowl of Soma. It is an excellent dish for cooling and calming down excess Pitta and Vata in your body. Each spoonful unfolds previously unnoticed nuances of flavor and creates a moment of peace in your system. It is easy to digest but nourishing enough to make for a light dinner when you don't have much of an appetite. If your fennel bulb came with stalks and fronds, they fit perfectly into this recipe—slice them up and use them. The taro root is the secret behind the velvety, creamy texture of this soup; see my Note below if you don't have taro on hand.

This wholesome, delectable, ivory-color soup goes well with Plain Basmati Rice (page 64), Vegetable Bread (page 70), and many more.

1 tablespoon ghee or olive oil

1 teaspoon slivered fresh ginger

1 teaspoon ground fennel seeds

1 teaspoon ground coriander

Tiny pinch of asafoetida

4 cups thinly sliced fennel bulb (2 medium bulbs with or without fronds)

1 medium taro root, peeled and thinly sliced (about ½ cup)

1 teaspoon salt, or to taste

2 teaspoons fresh lime juice, or to taste

GARNISHES

Freshly ground black pepper

Olive oil

4 teaspoons minced fresh dill or fennel frond leaves

FOR VATA OR PITTA BALANCING: Enjoy as is.

FOR KAPHA BALANCING: In Step 1, add 1 small green seeded and minced Indian or Thai chile with the ginger.

1. Melt the ghee in a 4-quart saucepan over medium-low heat. Add the ginger, ground fennel, coriander, and asafoetida, and toast for 10 seconds, then stir in the sliced fennel and taro. Cover and sweat the vegetables, stirring occasionally, for 5 minutes. Add 4 cups water and the salt. Bring the soup to a boil, then cover, lower the heat, and simmer for 10 to 15 minutes, until the vegetables are tender. Set the pot aside uncovered to let the soup cool down a bit.

2. Using a blender, puree the soup to a smooth, creamy consistency. Transfer it back to the saucepan, and gently heat the soup to serving temperature. Stir in the lime juice.

3. Serve hot. Garnish each individual bowl with a few turns of the peppermill, a drizzle of olive oil, and a sprinkle of dill.

VARIATION: To add protein, in a separate small saucepan, cook ½ cup chana dal (soaked in water overnight and rinsed) with 3 cups water for 45 minutes, or until the chana is soft and starts to break apart. Season the cooked chana with ½ teaspoon salt. When adding the lime juice in Step 2, fold in the chana and a little bit of its cooking liquid into the blended soup. The chana will give the soup a pleasant chunky texture.

NOTE: If you do not have taro root, mix 1 tablespoon arrowroot powder with 1 tablespoon water, and add it to the soup in Step 2, before blending.

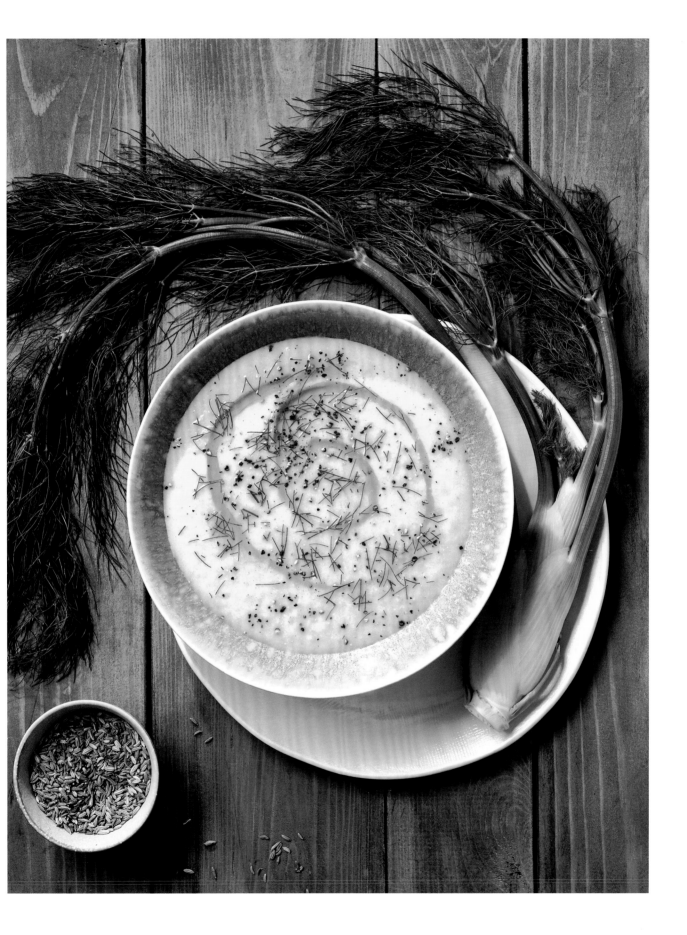

TUBERS, RHIZOMES, AND ROOTS

examples:

tubers

potatoes • taro • jicama • sunchokes •
sweet potatoes • yams • nagaimo

rhizomes

ginger • galangal • turmeric •
lotus root • fingerroot

roots

beets • carrots • radishes •
celery root • parsnips • rutabaga •
turnips • yucca • burdock

Ayurveda lists two groups of root vegetables: tubers and rhizomes (*kanda*) and roots (*mula*).

Although tubers, rhizomes, and roots are all root vegetables, they are classified separately by their underground growth patterns. Picture the aboveground and underground portion of any of these plants: with tubers, one plant will yield a few separate vegetables (think of potatoes); with roots, one plant will yield one vegetable (think of carrots); and a rhizome plant will yield multiple rootstalks, grown horizontally (think of ginger). Two often confused tubers are yams and sweet potatoes. Yams have a brown or black colored rough skin, with rounded ends, and sweet potatoes have lighter colored softer skins, with tapered ends.

Root vegetables are available year-round. They carry a lot of earthy energy, not only because they grow underground but also because they are dense, sweet, and heavy. No wonder we crave them in the cold weather! Since roots are among the hardest to digest vegetables, avoid eating them if you're feeling very weak.

Choose firm roots, and avoid any with undesirable cracks, soft spots, or mold. Always store your roots in a cool and dark place. In her classic book *The New Whole Foods Encyclopedia*, Rebecca Wood offers helpful advice on how to store roots:

"Most roots store best in the refrigerator for several weeks, but they are best within a few days of harvest. Packed in sand, roots hold in a root cellar for several months. Bright greens attached to a turnip or other root vegetable are a welcome sign of freshness. Home from the store, separate greens from roots at the leaf base, but do not cut into the root itself. Leaves left attached to a root draw moisture and flavor from it."

CARROTS

I love carrots because they are available anywhere in the world all year round, and they are inexpensive, delicious, and beautiful. People have cooked with carrots for thousands of years, and the ancient Ayurveda writers recognized carrots for their healing properties, including the use of carrot seeds in remedies to heal inflammation and fresh wounds. The seeds are also aphrodisiac, but pregnant women should not consume them due to a risk of miscarriage.

BOTANICAL NAME ● *Daucus Carota Linn.*

SANSKRIT NAME ● *Grinjanam, Garjar*

AYURVEDIC ATTRIBUTES

TASTE ● sweet, bitter

QUALITIES ● light to digest, unctuous, easy to absorb

METABOLIC EFFECT ● mildly heating

POST-DIGESTIVE EFFECT ● sweet

DOSHA EFFECTS ● pacifies Vata, Pitta, and Kapha

HEALING BENEFITS ● stimulates appetite, is diuretic, reduces flatulence, reverses brain and nerve weakness

SOURCING

● Carrots come in several varieties and colors. Whenever available, choose smaller, freshly picked carrots with green tops—these are the most flavorful and sweet.

SEASON

● Although their harvest season takes place from spring to fall, carrots are available throughout the year because they store well during the winter.

DIGESTIBILITY

● Carrots are high in lectins and therefore digest best when cooked, although it's okay to use a small amount of raw carrot for salads or fresh juice blends.

● Ayurveda's recommended dose of fresh carrot juice is 20 to 40 milliliters (0.7 to 1.4 ounces). This may sound like very little, but the small dose guarantees proper absorption. To better handle the natural sugar in the carrot juice, you may dilute it with a little spring water.

COOKING TIPS

● Carrots are great steamed, roasted, boiled, braised, sautéed, and caramelized.

● Use a spiralizer or a peeler to make carrot noodles and ribbons for an interesting presentation.

EAT CARROTS WHEN YOU NEED TO

● build strength and stamina,

● increase appetite,

● calm your brain and nerves,

● reduce flatulence,

● get over a cough, and/or

● strengthen your eyes.

roasted carrot tahini sauce

MAKES about 1¼ cups ● PREP: 10 minutes ● BAKE: 15 minutes ● GF, DF ●
Photograph on pages 195 and 250

This recipe is by Federica Norreri, a dear friend and a graduate of our Ayurvedic Nutrition and Culinary Training. She presented it as a side dish to her Savory Waffles—both dishes are fabulous and have been on the menu at Divya's Kitchen since day one.

The bright yellow color captures the eye, and the sauce's pungency pinches the tongue as the sweetness of the roasted carrots and the tartness of the lime juice unfold on your palate. This has become my substitute for mustard. Serve it with Sunflower-Beet Hummus (page 194), Braised Purple Cabbage (page 117), or as a sidekick to Broccoli Rabe and Beets with Saffron Almonds (page 102). It also makes a great dip for any crackers and dehydrated vegetable chips.

½ pound orange carrots, peeled and cut into ½-inch cubes

2 teaspoons olive oil

¼ cup roasted tahini

2 tablespoons fresh lime juice

1 teaspoon Za'atar (page 234)

1 green Indian or Thai chile, seeded

½ teaspoon salt, or to taste

1. Preheat the oven to 400°F. Line a small sheet pan with parchment paper (or use a glass baking dish without parchment).

2. Coat the carrots with the olive oil, spread them on the prepared dish, and roast for 15 minutes, or until the carrots have softened and lightly browned. Let the roasted carrots cool down to warm or room temperature.

3. In a blender, combine the roasted carrots, tahini, lime juice, Za'atar, chile, and ½ cup water, and blend until smooth. Check the consistency—you're looking for smooth and creamy and easy to pour. If it's too thick, add more water little by little until the sauce reaches this texture.

4. Refrigerate in an airtight container for up to three days. You might need to add a little more water to thin the refrigerated sauce.

roasted sweet potatoes

SERVES 2 to 3 ● **PREP:** 10 minutes ● **ROAST:** about 30 minutes ● **GF, DF** ● **FALL-WINTER**

This is another beloved side dish from the menu at Divya's Kitchen that is so simple to prepare yet so nourishing and satisfying, especially during the cold weather. There is something so comforting when you bite on a warm, slightly crusty orange sweet potato: it exudes a perfume-like aroma of spices, and it delightfully contrasts with the crunch of the toasted pecans and the red hue and tart flavor of the cranberries.

Although called "potatoes," sweet potatoes are not nightshades. And because they are low glycemic, they are an excellent way to satisfy a sweet craving without having to worry about spiking your blood sugar.

Roasted Sweet Potatoes will help you keep warm and grounded. They go well with Steamed Kale Salad (page 109), Braised Purple Cabbage (page 117), Sautéed Bitter Melon (page 135), Green Tahini Sauce (page 219), and more.

2 tablespoons melted ghee or coconut oil, plus more for greasing the pan

1 pound sweet potatoes (Garnet yams are a good choice), peeled and cut into ¾-inch cubes (about 4 cups)

1 teaspoon Sweet Masala #2 (page 234)

GARNISHES

2 tablespoons dried cranberries

2 tablespoons chopped toasted pecans

1. Preheat the oven to 400°F. Grease a 9 x 13-inch baking sheet with ghee or coconut oil.

2. In a large bowl, mix the ghee, sweet potatoes, and masala. Spread them onto the baking sheet, making sure to leave some space between the pieces.

3. Roast the sweet potatoes, stirring every 10 minutes, for about 30 minutes, until the sweet potatoes are soft and have a light golden crust.

4. Heat a skillet over medium-low heat. Add the pecans and toast them until they darken a shade. Transfer them to a small bowl and reserve for garnishing.

5. Garnish each serving with dried cranberries and toasted pecans. Serve hot.

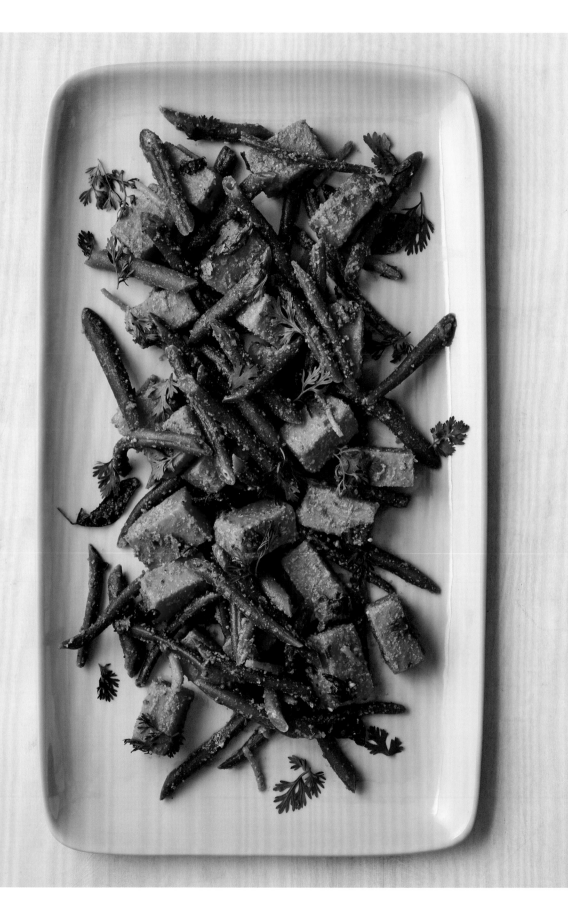

sweet potato and green bean salad

SERVES 3 to 4 • PREP: 20 minutes • COOK: 15 minutes • GF, DF • FALL-WINTER

Here is a balancing salad for the fall-winter season, when raw lettuce salads feel too cold and airy. I like how the seasonings lend a kick of heat to the grounding and satiating vegetables and create a sense of expansion within the body. Try this combination of spices, nuts, and seeds with other steamed vegetables: parsnips and kale; beets and carrots; baby turnips, carrots, and spinach, to name a few.

Sweet Potato and Green Bean Salad goes well with Adzuki Bean and Red Lentil Patties (page 84), Plain Basmati Rice (page 64), Lime Rice Pilaf (page 65), Cauliflower Soup with Almond Cream (page 120), and more.

2 cups peeled and cut sweet potatoes (½- by 1-inch pieces)

2 cups trimmed and cut (2 inches long) green beans

1 tablespoon cashew pieces or sunflower seeds

1½ teaspoons white sesame seeds

1 tablespoon toasted sesame oil

1 green Indian or Thai chile, seeded and minced

1 tablespoon peeled and thinly julienned fresh ginger

6 fresh curry leaves

½ teaspoon salt

½ teaspoon Protein Digestive Masala (page 233)

Tiny pinch of asafoetida

2 tablespoons fresh lime juice

¼ cup loosely packed fresh cilantro leaves

FOR VATA BALANCING: Reduce or omit the chile.

FOR PITTA BALANCING: Omit the chile and asafoetida.

FOR KAPHA BALANCING: Enjoy as is.

1. Steam the sweet potatoes and green beans in a steamer basket over medium heat for 10 to 15 minutes, until the vegetables are tender yet retain their vibrant colors. Rinse them under cold water and drain well. Transfer to a large bowl.

2. While the vegetables are steaming, dry-toast the cashew pieces and sesame seeds in a small skillet over medium-low heat, shaking frequently to allow the nuts and seeds to brown slightly. Set aside to cool. Powder the toasted ingredients in a spice grinder.

3. In a small skillet, heat the sesame oil over medium heat. Add the chile, ginger, curry leaves, salt, masala, and asafoetida, and toast for about 10 seconds to help the spices activate their aromas, then turn off the heat.

4. Pour the hot seasonings over the steamed vegetables. Add the lime juice and cilantro, and sprinkle the powdered cashew-sesame mixture on top. Toss gently to combine. Serve at room temperature.

TARO ROOT

Taro is one of the earliest cultivated tubers on earth. It is prominent in the culinary cultures of the Pacific, but it also grows in the north. In the landscaping of New York City, taro serves as a decorative plant because of its beautiful philodendron-like greenery.

I first tasted taro in Vrindavan, India, where it is known as *arbi*. On the spiritual holiday of Radhashtami, every household in town would make a taro preparation and take it to a temple.

Taro is called "potato of the tropics," but it is not a nightshade vegetable; that's why I use it as a potato substitute. When swapping taro for potato, keep in mind that taro is a little pastier and stickier in texture. Taro surpasses potato in taste, nutrition, and medicinal benefits, and it is highly valued in Shaka Vansiya Ayurveda as a pre-biotic. With its slippery nature, taro serves as a binder of toxins. In the words of Dr. Marianne Teitelbaum, taro is the "packaging and shipping" of toxins—it binds them together and drives them out of the body, making it an important ingredient in detox.

BOTANICAL NAME • *Colocasia esculenta*
SANSKRIT NAME • *Alooki*

AYURVEDIC ATTRIBUTES

TASTE • sweet

QUALITIES • heavy to digest, gooey, sticky

METABOLIC EFFECT • cooling (some varieties are warming)

POST-DIGESTIVE EFFECT • sweet

DOSHA EFFECTS • reduces Vata and Pitta, increases Kapha

HEALING BENEFITS • relieves inflammation in the lungs, heals the lining of the small and large intestines

SOURCING

- Depending on where in the world you live, you will find taro at a farmers market or at an Indian or Asian grocery store. It might be listed as one of its international names: *albi, arwi, dasheen,* or *eddo*. If you can't find taro, look for one of its close cousins: yautia, malanga, nagaimo, or even yucca.
- There are two main types of taro: a very large one (common in Hawaii) and a smaller potato-size one, with a brown and hairy skin. I use the small ones because they are easier to digest.

DIGESTIBILITY

- Always peel and cook taro root to minimize the calcium oxalate content found in its skin.
- Vaidya Mishra recommended that we eat taro at least twice a week (daily is also fine) to benefit from its binding properties. To make taro more Kapha balancing, add black pepper, chile, or ginger to the recipe.

COOKING TIPS

- Before washing taro root, peel, slice off any brown spots, and chop it—water makes the vegetable slippery and harder to cut.
- Cook taro until it is completely done and tender. A crunchy, half-cooked taro will produce *ama*.
- Mashed taro is a delicious substitute for mashed potatoes.
- These cooking methods work well with taro: stewing, roasting, braising, steaming, boiling.

EAT TARO ROOT WHEN YOU NEED TO

- reduce symptoms of rheumatoid arthritis,
- lower high blood pressure,
- ease body cramps,
- thicken your hair,
- prevent bone loss,
- stimulate circulation,
- improve your gut microbiome, and/or
- detox.

celery root and taro pancakes

MAKES nine 3½-inch wide pancakes ● PREP: 40 minutes ● COOK: 30 to 40 minutes ● GF, DF ●
FALL-WINTER

Potato pancakes are present in practically every European cuisine, including Bulgarian. Growing up, I remember my dad making patatnik with grated potatoes and feta cheese—it was so yummy! You might have memories of Jewish latkes, Irish boxty, or Czech bramboraky. This is my potato-free version of the popular pancakes, inspired by a similar recipe in Miriam Kasin Hospodar's *Heaven's Banquet*.

These pancakes are beautifully browned and so delicious. Sweet and savory, with a subtle nutty tone of the roots' earthiness—I would enjoy them anytime, but they feel especially balancing in the cold weather. The taro not only enhances the taste but also replaces an egg's binding effect.

Much more nutritious and flavorful than their potato cousins, Celery Root and Taro Pancakes draw attention and win praise every time we serve them at our cooking classes and events. Cashew Sour Cream (page 186), Green Tahini Sauce (page 219), Basil-Parsley Pesto (page 217), or Ayurvedic "Ketchup" (page 173) are sauce ideas to accompany these pancakes.

1 cup quinoa flakes

3 cups peeled and medium-grated celery root (from 2 large pieces)

1 cup peeled and medium-grated taro root (from 2 medium pieces)

¼ cup fresh parsley leaves, minced

¼ cup fresh basil leaves, chopped

2 tablespoons (12 grams) oat flour

1 teaspoon salt

½ teaspoon ground turmeric

½ teaspoon freshly ground black pepper

2 tablespoons fresh lime juice

3 tablespoons ghee or coconut oil for panfrying

FOR VATA OR PITTA BALANCING: Enjoy as is.

FOR KAPHA BALANCING: Serve with a hot sauce, or add 1 seeded and minced green Indian or Thai chile with the parsley in Step 2.

1. Place the quinoa flakes in a small bowl, add ½ cup water, and fluff with your fingers to make the flakes slightly moist and plump (they should not be dripping wet).

2. In a large bowl, toss together the celery root, taro, parsley, and basil. Fold in the quinoa flakes, oat flour, salt, turmeric, and pepper and mix well. Stir in ¼ cup water and the lime juice.

3. Wet your hands and shape the mixture into 9 equal balls, each about 2 inches in diameter. Of course, you can vary the size, smaller or bigger, according to your liking.

4. Heat 2 tablespoons of the ghee in a cast-iron griddle over medium-low heat. Shape each ball into a 3½-inch-wide and ⅓-inch-thick patty, and place it onto the hot griddle; repeat with the remaining balls to fill the griddle. Panfry, turning them with a sharp metal spatula, until each side is golden brown and slightly crispy, 7 to 10 minutes per side. You want to make sure that the middle layer of the pancakes is cooked—that the vegetables are not crunchy. Add more ghee to moisten the griddle and regulate the heat as you go—if

your pan starts to smoke, lower the heat. Lay the cooked pancakes on a sheet pan or large platter.

5. Serve immediately with your sauce of choice. If you're not serving them right away, keep the pancakes warm in the oven between 175°F and 200°F.

VARIATIONS: If you cannot find taro root, substitute it with 2 extra cups of grated celery root or parsnips. Add 1 tablespoon arrowroot powder and 1 more tablespoon oat flour in Step 2.

Replace all or half of the quinoa flakes with almond meal (the remaining pulp from making almond milk).

CELERY ROOT

Celery root (a.k.a. celeriac, celery knob) is a bit messy to work with. It's worth the effort, though, as this cold weather vegetable nourishes us with potassium and phosphorus and helps us clear ama.

BOTANICAL NAME ● *Apium graveolens*

SANSKRIT NAME ● unknown

AYURVEDIC ATTRIBUTES

TASTE ● sweet, slightly bitter and sour

QUALITIES ● heavy, rough

METABOLIC EFFECT ● cooling

POST-DIGESTIVE EFFECT ● sweet or sour

DOSHA EFFECTS ● balances all three doshas

HEALING BENEFITS ● supports the lymphatic, nervous, digestive, and urinary systems

SOURCING

● Buy celery root (ideally with its stems and leaves attached) from the farmers market or grocery store. Select small and firm knobs. Before refrigerating, cut off the roots from the stems and store them separately.

SEASON

● Celery root is seasonal in the fall, winter, and early spring.

DIGESTIBILITY

● A crunchy celery root can increase Vata and bloating; that's why I recommend cooking it until soft but not mushy.

● Good digestive and flavor seasonings include caraway seeds, fennel seeds, lime juice, parsley, thyme, and nutmeg.

COOKING TIPS

● The messy part of working with celeriac is its knobbiness and dirt-filled crevices. I handle this by peeling the root with a knife.

● Use a small amount of the slightly bitter celery root stems and greens in soups and stews.

● You can stew, sauté, stir-fry, puree, braise, marinate, or roast celery root.

EAT CELERY ROOT WHEN YOU NEED TO

● lower blood pressure,

● reduce inflammation,

● lose weight,

● relieve indigestion, and/or

● eliminate kidney stones.

Opposite: Celery Root and Taro Pancakes, Green Tahini Sauce

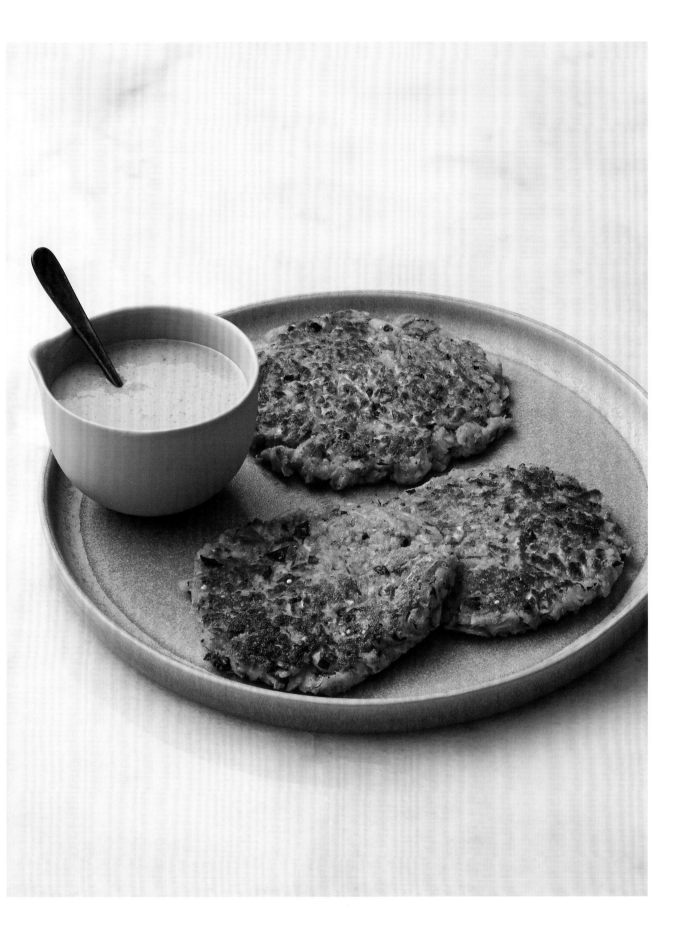

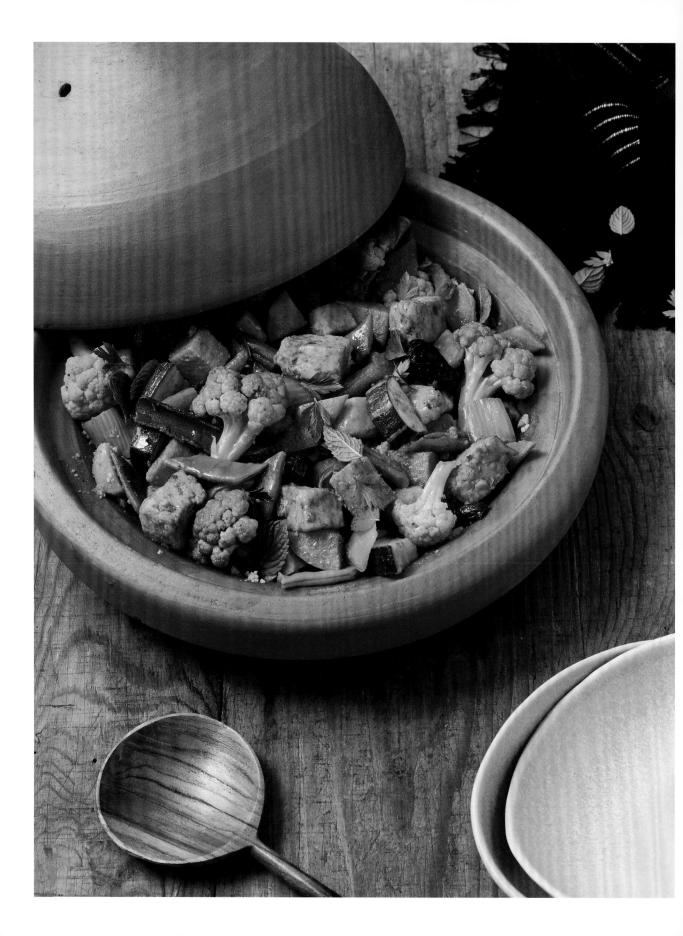

moroccan-style vegetable tagine

SERVES 4 to 6 ● **PREP:** 20 minutes (with already made paneer cheese) ● **COOK:** 25 minutes ●
GF, DF OPTION ● **YEAR-ROUND**

I'm very grateful to my friend and colleague Michael Burdi for introducing me to Moroccan and Middle Eastern cuisines. With the richness of spices and clay-pot cooking methods, a lot of their dishes come very close to the Ayurvedic principles of cooking.

Tagine is the name of the traditional earthen pot that this dish is cooked in. The dome-shaped lid helps circulate all steam condensation back to the bottom of the pot, thus allowing the food to cook with minimally added water. The main trick is to cook it slowly.

This dish has such bright, warm colors—a joyful display of Moroccan art. You can serve it with Plain Basmati Rice (page 64) or cooked millet instead of the traditional couscous (less nutritious) or with flatbread. A lime pickle is a delicious condiment with this dish.

5 pitted prunes

¾ teaspoon coriander seeds

½ teaspoon cumin seeds

2 tablespoons ghee

½ cup diced (¼-inch) fennel bulb

1 tablespoon minced fresh ginger

2¾-inch cinnamon stick

⅛ teaspoon asafoetida

10 ounces (1½ cups) pressed paneer cheese (page 205; made from ½ gallon milk; optional), cut into ¾-inch cubes

2 teaspoons salt

¼ teaspoon paprika (optional)

¼ teaspoon ground turmeric

⅛ teaspoon saffron strands

2½ pounds vegetables, cut into ¾-inch pieces: taro root, cauliflower, green beans, zucchini, and sweet potato (about 1 cup of each)

8 pitted green or black olives, cut in half

GARNISHES

Olive oil

2 tablespoons chopped fresh parsley

1 tablespoon chopped fresh mint leaves

FOR VATA OR PITTA BALANCING: Enjoy as is.

FOR KAPHA BALANCING: Add 1 or 2 seeded and minced green Indian or Thai chiles with the spices in Step 3.

1. Soak the prunes in a bowl with hot water for 10 minutes, then drain.

2. Meanwhile, in an electric spice grinder, grind the coriander and cumin seeds to a powder.

3. Heat the ghee in a large tagine pot or sauté pan over medium heat. Add the fennel, ginger, cinnamon, and asafoetida, lower the heat to medium-low, and sauté for 5 minutes. Add the paneer, salt, ground coriander and cumin, paprika, turmeric, and saffron. Sauté for 5 more minutes, or until the cheese cubes have softened and are coated in the seasonings.

4. Fold in the vegetables, olives, prunes, and 1 cup hot water. Cover, decrease the heat to low, and simmer, shaking occasionally, until the vegetables are tender but not mushy, about 15 minutes.

5. Garnish each serving with a drizzle of olive oil and a sprinkle of parsley and mint. Serve hot.

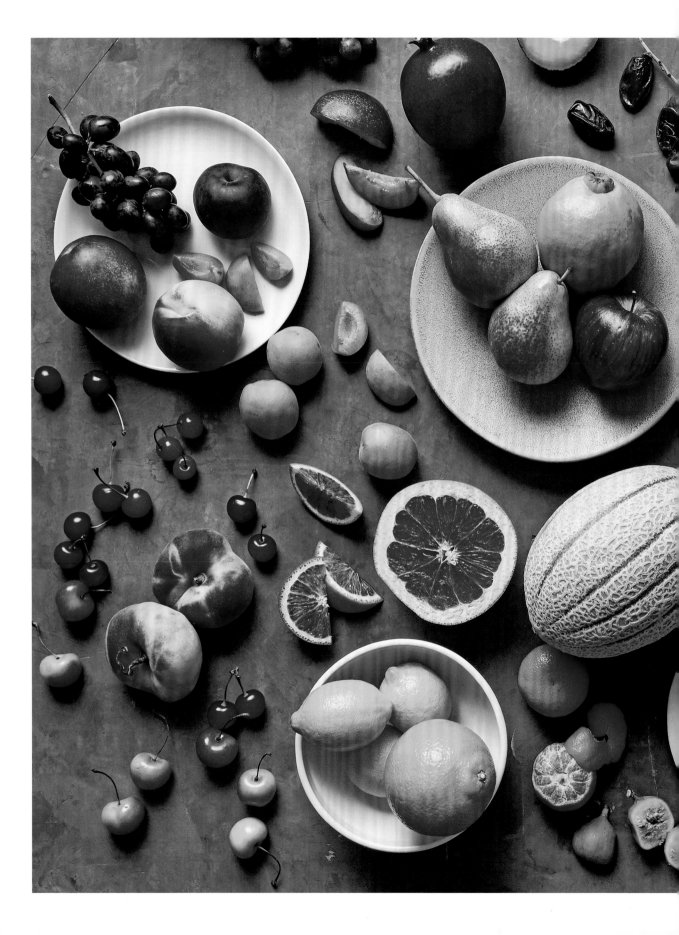

FRUITS

FRUITS

examples:

pome fruits
apples • pears • quince

stone fruits
peaches • apricots • cherries
plums • prunes

berry fruits
blueberries • raspberries • strawberries
blackberries • grapes • pomegranates

citrus
oranges • lemons • limes • grapefruits •
mandarins • tangerines

melons
watermelon • cantaloupe • honeydew

tropical and subtropical fruits
bananas • pineapple • papaya •
dates • tamarind • mango • avocado •
kiwi • lychee

medicinal
wild berries • amla • elderberry • rose hips

Unlike grains, legumes, and most vegetables, fruits can easily be eaten raw. They are a good source of natural sugars, minerals, fiber, and antioxidants, and they give us a quick boost of energy. Most varieties are light to digest and can make a pleasant meal by themselves, especially in warm weather. A bowl of sweet and juicy fruit on a hot day is most refreshing.

I try to plan my family trips to Bulgaria in the summer so that I can take advantage of its seasonal fruit opulence. It must be something about the soil and the climate that makes Bulgarian fruits so flavorful and delicious—the kind of taste I still long to experience in the US. My mom loves to grow an assortment of fruits that reach their peak sweetness in chronological order throughout the summer. First appear the strawberries and the cherries, then blush the peaches and apricots; August is the month for heavenly figs, and early September calls for harvesting her multiple sorts of apples, pears, plums, prunes, and grapes. Later in the fall, Mom would pick kiwis from the overhead yard vines that provided her shade all summer, and finally, the bright red pomegranates announce the end of the year's warm days.

The ancient Ayurvedic textbooks classify fruits as *phala-varga* and describe about seventy-five varieties (including nuts, which are considered shell fruits), many of which are extinct today. Back then, grapes and raisins, followed by pomegranate, amla, and mangoes were considered the best of fruit. I am sure that if those wise authors were able to travel and examine fruits from around the world today, they would still be capable of describing the best of each region. In general, the juicer the fruit, the more medicinal its attributes.

Based on some Ayurvedic texts and my culinary experience, here are some tips on how to get the most out of your fruit consumption:

- Favor naturally ripened, local, organic, seasonal, and succulent fruit.

- Avoid fruits that have been affected by birds, animals, or insects.

- Store firm and almost-ripe fruit at room temperature, and once matured, refrigerate it.

- For Vata balancing: eat sweet, tart, or cooked fruit—ideally one type at a time, in a small amount.

- For Pitta balancing: eat sweet and juicy fruit; larger amounts are okay.

- For Kapha balancing: eat mildly sweet and tart fruit, not very watery or oily; enjoy in small amounts; dried fruit is great if your Vata functions are in good shape.

It's best to eat fruit on its own, ideally between meals (as a snack) or 30 minutes before lunch. Do not eat raw fruit for dessert, as its combination with other foods tends to create confusion and fermentation in the stomach, leading to bloating and gas. Do not eat fruit late at night because it is too heavy for your diminishing *agni*.

Exceptions to the above guidelines are small amounts of papaya, pineapple, and pomegranate with your lunch meal. Their unique digestive enzymes do not upset the stomach.

Cooked fruit digests differently from raw fruit, and it is OK to eat with other foods or in a meal. It is also preferred over raw fruit for people with weak digestion.

Sprinkle a pinch of black salt on your raw, fresh fruit to enhance taste and digestibility.

Two popular fruit-related diets in our modern times are fruitarian and juicing. Ayurveda warns us that an all-fruit diet could be temporarily suited for a high Pitta person who lives in a warm climate and does not do intensive physical labor. In all other cases, a long-term fruitarian diet would gradually create deep dosha imbalances.

The ancient texts mention fruit juices, such as grape and pomegranate, but the recommended quantity is only 50 to 100 milliliters at a time. Back to our discussion on portioning on page 31, juice is another source of nourishment we tend to overdo in the West. Try fresh juice in small doses— this will allow you to better absorb its nutrients. If you tend to have blood sugar issues or you're serving it to children, dilute the fruit juice with water to a 50:50 ratio. I like to juice a small piece of ginger with my very sweet fruit juices, such as grapes, to enhance their digestibility.

APPLES

Apple picking is one of my favorite activities in my mom's garden. In early September, her trees bend their branches with the heavy fruit as if bowing down and submissively requesting, "Please pick us."

With over seventy-five hundred cultivars, apples are the most widely grown fruit on the planet. Apples are so versatile—we use them for cooking, juicing, or making pectin, cider, vinegar, and alcohol.

BOTANICAL NAME • *Pyrus malus, malus domestica*

SANSKRIT NAME • *Seva*

AYURVEDIC ATTRIBUTES

TASTE • astringent, sweet

QUALITIES • heavy to digest

METABOLIC EFFECT: • cooling

POST-DIGESTIVE EFFECT • sweet

DOSHA EFFECTS • raw apples are best for balancing Pitta and Kapha; cooked apples are best suited for Vata

HEALING BENEFITS • enhances taste; increases semen amount; strengthens the heart, lungs, spleen, stomach, and large intestine

SOURCING

- Apples are easily available anywhere in the world. Fuji and Granny Smith are some of the most enduring varieties. This pome fruit is among the most chemically treated foods; therefore it is best to buy it organic. Apples of excellent quality are bruise-free, firm, and have their stem attached.

SEASON

- Even though harvested in the early fall, apples store well through the winter and are considered seasonal during the cold months, up until March.

DIGESTIBILITY

- Raw, unpeeled apples can increase *Vata* and cause gas and bloating. For easier digestion, peel the apple and eat it alone, as a snack (do not mix with other food). Or, cook the apple—in this case, you can mix it with other food.

- Eat a raw apple an hour or so after lunch to clean your tongue and teeth and support regularity with your bowel movements.

- Don't eat apples at night.

COOKING TIPS

- I like the sweet-tart apple varieties (Fuji, Pink Lady, Gala, Opal) for cooking because they better retain their shape.

- Sweet apples (McIntosh, Elstar, Gravenstein) tend to cook into a softer consistency—they work well for applesauce.

- Eat a cooked apple first thing in the morning to enhance your *agni* and clean your gut (see my recipe for Cooked Apple Pre-Breakfast in *What to Eat for How You Feel*).

EAT AN APPLE WHEN YOU NEED TO

- relieve constipation,
- reduce excessive salivation,
- get rid of cold sores in the mouth, and/or
- lower bad cholesterol.

cooked apple-beet smoothie

SERVES 1 to 2 ● **PREP:** 10 minutes ● **COOK:** 10 minutes ● **GF, DF** ● **FALL**

I created this recipe for my friend Kristen, who came to me crying, "Everything feels stuck in my stomach; I'm in pain and nauseous. I react to almost everything I eat. I don't know what to eat!" Her pulse indicated that her digestive fire was very low and her gallbladder and liver were sluggish, so I made this smoothie for her and gave her the recipe. Within an hour, her pain had subsided and things started moving. After three days of drinking it first thing in the morning, she felt "infinitely better." My smoothie hit the spot!

A lot of the common digestive problems and food allergies we experience today are due to congested bile. It is very important to take care of our liver and gallbladder and to ensure healthy bile production and flow. Ayurveda offers many solutions to keep our bile thin and moving. Ayurveda also warns us against the foods and eating habits that tend to congest our bile (see page 33).

This ruby-colored smoothie is fantastic for improving digestion by flushing out bile sludge and for thinning congested bile. For being such an effective blood builder, this recipe is very delicious! There are a couple of contraindications for using this recipe—see Notes.

Enjoy a cup of this smoothie first thing in the morning, as a pre-breakfast, or as an afternoon snack.

1 small red beet, peeled and thinly sliced (about ½ cup)

1 tablespoon raisins

1-inch piece cinnamon stick

2 teaspoons minced fresh ginger

½ teaspoon fennel seeds

¼ teaspoon fenugreek seeds

⅛ teaspoon salt

1 medium Granny Smith apple

FOR PITTA BALANCING: Omit the ginger.

FOR VATA OR KAPHA BALANCING: Enjoy as is.

1. In a small saucepan, combine 1½ cups water, the beets, raisins, cinnamon stick, ginger, fennel seeds, fenugreek seeds, and salt. Cover and bring to a boil over medium-high heat, then lower the heat and simmer for 3 minutes, or until the beet slices are half-cooked.

2. Meanwhile, peel, core, and chop the apple.

3. Add the apple to the pan and continue to simmer, covered, until the apple and beets are fully cooked, about 3 minutes.

4. Set aside uncovered to let cool to warm. Remove the cinnamon stick.

5. Transfer to a blender, and blend until smooth. Add more water if you like a thinner consistency. Enjoy warm or at room temperature.

VARIATION: Add 2 tablespoons fresh orange juice in Step 5.

NOTES: If you have been diagnosed with gallstones, drink this smoothie only under the supervision of a medical doctor or Ayurvedic practitioner, as your thinner and moving bile may push some gallstones into a bile duct, obstruct it, and cause serious problems.

Do not drink this smoothie if you have diarrhea.

PEARS

BOTANICAL NAME ● *Pyrus communis*

SANSKRIT NAME: ● *Tanka*

AYURVEDIC ATTRIBUTES

TASTE ● sweet, astringent

QUALITIES ● easy to digest

METABOLIC EFFECT ● cooling

POST-DIGESTIVE EFFECT ● sweet or pungent

DOSHA EFFECTS ● sweet and juicy pears mitigate all three doshas

HEALING BENEFITS ● aphrodisiac, diuretic

SOURCING

● Pears are easily available in most parts of the world. As with apples, this fruit is heavily treated with chemicals; therefore, buy it organic when possible. If your pears are hard, leave them to ripen at room temperature until they soften and become juicier; then refrigerate and use them within a few days.

SEASON

● The fall is when we harvest pears, but they store well through the winter, especially if you wrap them individually with paper and keep them in a single layer in a cool storage spot.

DIGESTIBILITY

● Peeled and cooked pears are easier to digest than unpeeled and raw.

● Cook pears with spices such as cinnamon, cloves, ginger, fennel, nutmeg, or star anise to make them more digestible.

● A sweet and juicy pear can instantly appease sharp, acidic digestion. It is also a good snack when you're hungry but can't yet eat a full meal.

COOKING TIPS

● The Bosc, Bartlett, and Anjou varieties are best for cooking because they retain their shape well.

● Swap your cooked morning apple with a pear for a change. It will provide you with the same digestive and cleansing effects. (See my recipe for Cooked Apple Pre-Breakfast in *What to Eat for How You Feel*).

EAT A PEAR WHEN YOU NEED TO

● stop diarrhea,

● increase appetite,

● ease abdominal cramps,

● relieve excessive thirst,

● stop bleeding gums,

● cool down quickly, and/or

● overcome a hangover (especially fresh pear juice).

CAUTION ● Do not eat pears if you suffer from sciatica, arthritis, diabetes, or dry cough.

apple-pear turnovers
with yacon "caramel" sauce

MAKES 6 large turnovers ● PREP: 45 minutes ● COOK: 35 minutes ● DF ● FALL-WINTER

There is something very enchanting about stuffed pastries, be it a samosa, empanada, spanakopita, apple strudel, or the filo-cheese banitza I grew up with—it's so hard to resist such treats! The trick to making them healthy is to use whole-grain flour, unrefined sweetener, and some spices for better digestion and flavor.

As with any stuffed dish, making these turnovers is a bit time-consuming, but you can stage the steps and keep the pastries refrigerated until you're ready to bake them. My turnover version looks more like an empanada than an American turnover (commonly made with puff pastry). The baked pastries brushed with maple syrup develop a thin crust, which makes the turnover crispy on the outside and soft on the inside, and the sauce adds a layer of moisture and caramel-like sweetness.

Serve Apple-Pear Turnovers with Yacon "Caramel" Sauce for breakfast, as a dessert, or include them in a picnic spread. I also like to travel with them because they are filling and easy to eat without making a lot of mess.

FILLING

1 tablespoon coconut oil or ghee

2-inch cinnamon stick

½ teaspoon kalonji seeds

¼ teaspoon ajwain seeds

1 teaspoon Sweet Masala #2 (page 234)

2 medium apples, peeled and diced into ⅓-inch pieces (about 2 cups)

2 pears, peeled and diced into ⅓-inch pieces (about 2 cups)

2 tablespoons raisins

3 tablespoons Sucanat or turbinado sugar

¼ cup finely chopped walnuts (optional)

DOUGH

1¼ cups (120 grams) sifted spelt flour

1 heaping cup (100 grams) sifted einkorn flour, plus more for dusting

1 tablespoon powdered sugar (see Note)

½ teaspoon salt

¼ teaspoon baking powder

¼ cup olive oil, melted coconut oil, or melted ghee, plus olive oil or coconut oil for the pan

½ cup buttermilk or boiling hot water

2 tablespoons maple syrup

YACON "CARAMEL" SAUCE

1 teaspoon arrowroot powder

⅓ cup yacon syrup

¼ teaspoon vanilla extract

CONTINUED

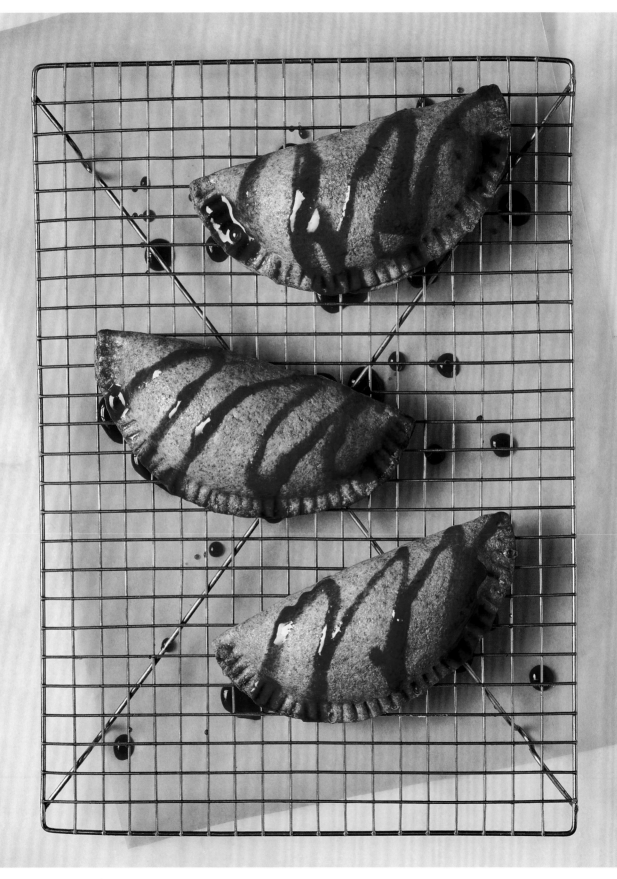

To make the filling:

1. Heat a medium sauté pan over medium-low heat, and add the coconut oil. Add the cinnamon stick, kalonji seeds, and ajwain seeds, and toast for 5 seconds, then add the masala. Stir in the apples, pears, and raisins. Once they start simmering, cover the pan and let the fruit sweat over low heat for about 10 minutes, until it is soft but not mushy. If your fruit starts sticking to the bottom of the pan, splash it with a little water. There should be no liquid around the cooked fruit; if that's the case, cook uncovered for a couple of minutes to evaporate it. Turn off the heat, and mix in the sugar and walnuts. Set aside to cool to room temperature.

To make the dough:

2. In a medium bowl, combine the spelt and einkorn flours, powdered sugar, salt, and baking powder, and mix well. Rub in the oil, then pour in the buttermilk, mix the dough, and shape it into a ball (if using hot water instead of buttermilk, you might want to use a disposable glove to tolerate the initial heat). The texture should be soft but not sticky.

3. Vigorously knead the dough for about 5 minutes, until it is smooth and bounces back from your touch. If the dough is too sticky, dust the kneading surface with einkorn flour as you continue to knead. Transfer the dough back into the bowl, cover it with a damp kitchen towel (not a paper towel!), and refrigerate for 15 minutes.

To assemble the turnovers:

4. Preheat the oven to 375°F. Line a half-size sheet pan with parchment paper or a silicone mat, and grease it with olive oil or coconut oil.

5. Divide the dough into 6 equal balls (about 76 grams each). After each is formed, keep it under the damp towel to prevent it from crusting.

6. Using your hands, roll one of the dough balls into a perfect ball. Using a rolling pin, roll the ball into a circle, about 2 millimeters thick and 6 inches in diameter. Place 2 tablespoons of the filling in one half of the circle and fold over the other half. Using your fingertips, press the overlapping edges together to seal the turnover. Make a pattern around the edge by pressing it with a fork or crimping it like a samosa (or whatever pattern you like). Place on the prepared sheet pan. Repeat this step to make the remaining turnovers.

7. Brush each turnover with maple syrup and place them in the oven. Bake for about 20 minutes, until the turnovers have a slight golden crust.

To make the sauce:

8. While the turnovers are baking, mix the arrowroot powder with 2 teaspoons water in a tiny bowl.

9. In a small saucepan, combine ½ cup water and the yacon syrup, and bring to a simmer. Add the arrowroot mixture, whisking it until the sauce thickens to a thin and smooth consistency (thinner than the consistency of the yacon syrup). Whisk in the vanilla and set aside.

10. Serve the Apple-Pear Turnovers warm, drizzled with the Yacon "Caramel" Sauce on top. I also like to serve extra sauce on the side because it is so delicious; you or your guests will inevitably ask for more.

NOTE: To make powdered sugar, grind raw cane sugar in a spice grinder until very fine.

HIBISCUS

When I lived in India, I saw hibiscus flowers growing in every garden. At that time, I never connected the beautiful red flowers of the garden shrub to the maroon dried petals I loved to make tea with. In India, hibiscus is regarded as a sacred flower. It is used in devotional ceremonies to Shri Ganesh, the personification of wisdom who destroys all obstacles and grants the achievement of one's goals.

BOTANICAL NAME • *Hibiscus rosa-sinensis Linn.*
SANSKRIT NAME • *Japa, Japa pushpa*

AYURVEDIC ATTRIBUTES

TASTE • astringent, sweet
QUALITIES • light, oily
METABOLIC EFFECT • cooling
POST-DIGESTIVE EFFECT • sweet
DOSHA EFFECTS • Tridoshic, but large amounts can imbalance Vata
HEALING BENEFITS • lowers high fever, stimulates hair growth, mitigates urinary disorders, prevents abnormal cell growth, lowers high blood pressure, facilitates weight loss, strengthens the immune system, prevents blood clots, strengthens women's reproductive system, reduces heavy menstrual flow, purifies the heart, physically and spiritually

COOKING TIPS

• Make a cold infusion by adding ¼ cup of dried hibiscus flowers to a jar and covering them with 4 cups of room temperature spring or filtered water. Let the herb steep overnight, then strain and sip slowly. For an extra Soma-like, cooling, and nurturing effect, leave the jar outside in the moonlight to steep.

CAUTION • Do not use if you are experiencing chills or severe Vata aggravation.

pineapple-hibiscus drink

MAKES 5 cups • **SOAK:** 8 hours or overnight •
PREP: 5 minutes (with already made juice) •
GF, DF • **YEAR-ROUND**

This is a favorite drink at Divya's Kitchen. Its beautiful ruby color and smooth texture are just so attractive. I recommend this drink not just for pleasure but also for its healing properties—it stimulates digestive enzymes, soothes the digestive tract, and delivers the many benefits of hibiscus and pineapple in a delicious way.

¼ cup dried hibiscus flowers

2½ cups fresh sweet pineapple juice (from 1 pineapple), strained

2 to 3 tablespoons maple syrup (optional, if the pineapple is not very sweet)

1. Place the hibiscus flowers in a 1-quart vessel and pour in 3 cups room temperature filtered or spring water. Cover and leave on the counter for at least 8 hours or overnight. Strain and reserve the liquid; discard the hibiscus.

2. Stir together the hibiscus water and pineapple juice. Taste and decide if you need to add the maple syrup for a pleasant sweetness. Enjoy at room temperature or slightly chilled. Store refrigerated for up to three days.

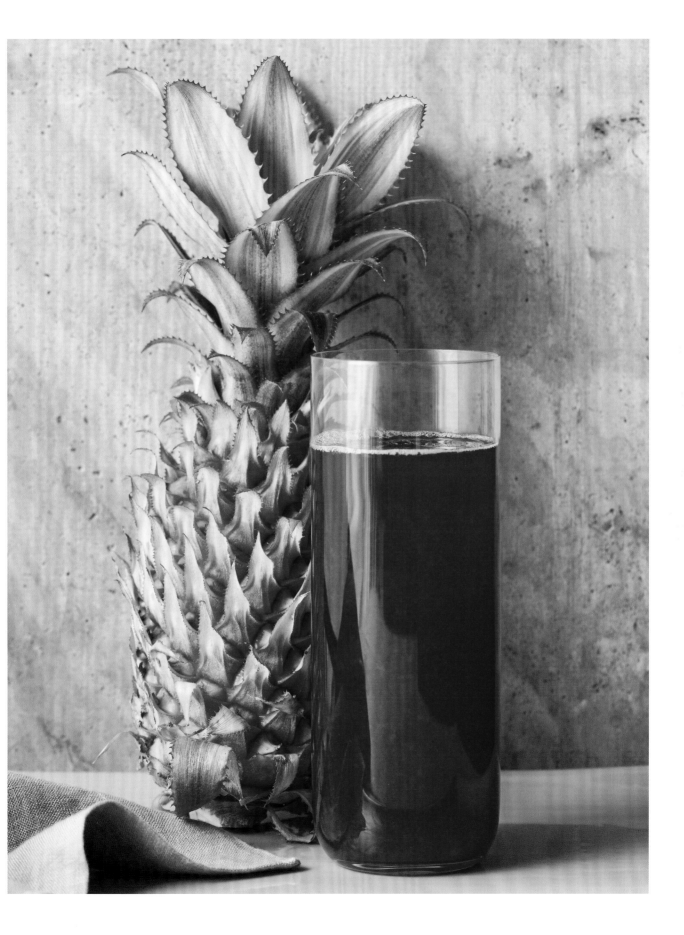

PINEAPPLE

A single fruit with a worldwide history, pineapple originated in Brazil and entered Europe and India in the seventeenth century. Today it is the third most cultivated tropical fruit in the world.

During my childhood years in Bulgaria, I tasted pineapple only in the form of canned juice. I loved it back then, and I relish it even more as a fresh beverage today. I find the fibrous, acidic flesh of the pineapple too agitating for my sensitive teeth, which is why I only consume it juiced. I adore fresh pineapple juice. What grabs me is the combination of the pleasant yellow color, exotic aroma, and sweet and slightly tart taste that, when savored in smooth sips, leaves a delicate coating in my mouth. I also appreciate how quickly pineapple improves my digestion.

Fresh pineapple juice is the most common therapeutic application of the fruit in Ayurveda.

BOTANICAL NAME ● *Ananas comosus*

SANSKRIT NAME ● *Ananas*

AYURVEDIC ATTRIBUTES

TASTE ● sweet (ripe), sour (unripe)

QUALITIES ● heavy, unctuous

METABOLIC EFFECT ● cooling (ripe), heating (unripe)

POST-DIGESTIVE EFFECT ● sweet

DOSHA EFFECTS ● pacifies Vata and Pitta

HEALING BENEFITS ● strengthens *agni,* serves as a mild laxative, helps with bleeding disorders

SOURCING

● Pineapple's famed sweetness and aroma build while the fruit is attached to the plant, and once disconnected, it will not get much sweeter. Unfortunately, most pineapple producers today pick their harvest before full maturation to prevent spoilage during transportation. Therefore, it is almost impossible to purchase a fully ripened and sweet pineapple outside of its growing habitat.

● At its prime, this cone-shaped fruit is of an orange-like color on the outside and a rich yellow on the inside (or light pink for the pink variety), and it exudes a sweet aroma at the base. It feels heavy, like a filled jug, when you hold it. Look for a firm fruit; discolored or soft spots indicate bruising.

● Avoid green, unripe pineapple because it is too sour and flavorless. You also don't want the overmature fruit because it is too mushy and tastes fermented. Canned pineapple is the least wholesome version of the fruit because it lacks *prana*.

● To store, cut off the leafy crown and invert the pineapple (bottom up) on the countertop for a couple of days—this will move sweetness from the base to the less-sweet crown. Ideally, enjoy the entire mature fruit the same day you cut into it because its flavor quickly diminishes once cut and refrigerated.

SEASON

● Pineapple is an herbaceous perennial plant. It is available all year long, but its peak season in the US is from April through July.

DIGESTIBILITY

● Being rich in manganese, vitamin C, and the digestive enzyme bromelain, pineapple is a marvelous prebiotic and digestive aid. It enhances *agni* and supports the breakdown of proteins and carbohydrates. This is one of the very few raw fruits that SV Ayurveda approves to mix with cooked food in a meal, especially for lunch.

● Avoid eating it at night because its tartness will agitate your Pitta and prevent you from falling asleep.

COOKING TIPS

- Pineapple is a fleshy, scale-coated fruit, and thus its peeled slices keep their shape when roasted, grilled, or baked. However, to benefit from its vitamin C and digestive enzymes, it is best to serve pineapple raw—in salads, chutneys, salsas, or drinks.
- To prevent sogginess in a salad, add it just before serving.
- Juice the pineapple (including its core) just before drinking it; enjoy the juice on its own or in small sips with lunch.
- Unlike most other ingredients that take on a gel-like texture when they're mixed with gelatin, agar-agar, or Irish moss, raw pineapple will not do this.

DRINK THE JUICE OF RIPE AND SWEET PINEAPPLE WHEN YOU NEED TO

- increase appetite,
- reverse constipation,
- clear heaviness in the stomach,
- cleanse *ama* from the gut,
- heal faster from jaundice,
- strengthen the heart,
- overcome a sore throat,
- relieve symptoms of bronchitis, and/or
- speed up childbirth labor.

CAUTION ● Do not eat pineapple during pregnancy (except when you reach your due date), because its purgative effects can induce a miscarriage or premature labor. Also avoid it if you struggle with hyperacidity.

TAMARIND

Years ago, when I lived in the holy town of Vrindavan, India, one of my favorite sites of pilgrimage was Imli Tala, on the banks of the Yamuna River. There is a small temple and, in the courtyard, a very old tamarind tree (*imli* is the Hindi word for "tamarind"). It used to spread its branches in all directions, as if to serve as the temple's guardian. I loved sitting under that tree and meditating because the saturated spiritual energy made it so easy for me to concentrate. At that time, the tamarind tree was my shelter; I was unaware of it as a source of food. As I deepened my Ayurveda studies, I experienced its magnificent taste and healing benefits.

Tamarind might be a foreign ingredient to you, so embrace the opportunity to connect with it and take advantage of its distinguished properties.

BOTANICAL NAME ● *Tamarindus indica*

SANSKRIT NAMES ● *Tintidik, Amlika*, and more

AYURVEDIC ATTRIBUTES (FOR RIPE, SWEET TAMARIND)

TASTE ● sour

QUALITIES ● heavy, dry

METABOLIC EFFECT ● slightly heating

POST-DIGESTIVE EFFECT ● sour

DOSHA EFFECTS ● balances the three doshas (the sour variety aggravates Pitta and Kapha and is constipating)

HEALING BENEFITS ● aids digestion, reduces heat in the blood, supports the liver and the heart (when cooked), serves as a prebiotic, lowers a fever, scrapes old toxins from the large intestine

CONTINUED

SOURCING

- The sweet-sour taste of this fruit varies between cultivars and ripeness. The best type is the sweet, ripe tamarind sold as whole pods. Fresh sweet tamarind is sold in health food stores, Indian and Asian markets, and online. I avoid tamarind paste because it is overly sour and gut irritating.

SEASON

- The tamarind tree grows in tropical climates, and its fruits ripen at different times of the year, depending on location. In Ayurveda, tamarind has been used in refreshing drinks during the summer, in sauces, desserts, and more. I like to use it all year round.

DIGESTIBILITY

- Sweet tamarind can be used raw, but it is best digested when briefly cooked. The pulp itself is very high in digestive enzymes and serves as a digestive, especially in dishes with high protein and fat.

COOKING TIPS

- In cooking, we only use the tamarind pulp, which is hidden in the fruit's pod. Below, I describe two ways to clean a tamarind pod so you can get to its pulp. The first step for both methods is to crack the outer shell and remove it and the hard strings around the pulp.

- For dry pulp: Use your fingertips to scrape away the soft and sticky pulp from the seeds and the skin that covers them (discard the seeds and skin). This is time-consuming, but the dry pulp stores in the refrigerator for up to two months.

- For wet pulp (paste): Cover the shelled tamarind with just enough boiling hot water, and let it soak for 10 to 20 minutes. Set a fine-mesh strainer above a bowl, and using a metal serving spoon, press the softened pulp through the strainer to separate the paste. You might have to add a little more water to the strainer to get all the pulp through. Refrigerate the tamarind paste for up to a week.

- I like using the dry pulp in my recipes because it gives a more accurate measurement, whereas the volume and water content of the paste varies.

- When adding chunks of tamarind pulp to a stew, use the dry pulp of 1 pod for two servings.

- Use tamarind pulp or paste in curries, soups, stews, drinks, dressings, or sauces. Or try it as a tomato replacement—it's sweet and tangy and can create a creamy base in a soup-like meal or condiment.

EAT RIPE, SWEET TAMARIND WHEN YOU NEED TO

- alleviate excessive thirst,
- increase appetite,
- strengthen the digestion of protein and fat,
- improve liver and colon functions,
- improve the absorption of nutrients,
- reverse constipation, and/or
- reduce morning sickness during pregnancy.

ayurvedic "ketchup"

MAKES about 1 cup ● PREP: 5 minutes (with already separated tamarind pulp) ● COOK: 15 minutes ●
GF, DF ● FALL-WINTER ● Photograph on pages 85 and 202

"Tomato-free ketchup? Really?!" This was my spontaneous reaction when I first saw this recipe in *Ayurvedic Cooking for Balance and Bliss*, by Vaidya R. K. Mishra and Rick Talcott. Years ago, I was avoiding tomatoes because of my chronic inflammatory disorder, and I was really missing the sweet and tangy pleasures of ketchup. Fortunately, Vaidya always knew how to give us healthier alternatives to our favorite "junk" foods. I think this sauce is as good as ketchup can get. It has the color, consistency, and flavors close to its popular counterpart but with significantly less acidic digestive effects; plus it gives you the rare health benefits of sweet tamarind.

Vaidya's recipe surprised me in yet another way: it uses vinegar! "But, Vaidya, you said, 'No vinegar because it is too acidic!'" I objected. Of course, Vaidya had a good reason. Not only did he want his version to closely resemble the traditional taste of ketchup but also to support our healing, rather than defy it. To me, this was an enlightening example of how a master makes an exception to the rule.

Serve Ayurvedic "Ketchup" with patties, pizza, pasta, cooked vegetables, breads, crackers, and baked fries. Please keep in mind that this recipe could be too heating for someone with a high Pitta imbalance.

¾ cup (4 ounces) dried cranberries

⅓ cup (2½ ounces) dry pulp from sweet Thai tamarind (or 1 cup tamarind-water paste)

1½ teaspoons Protein Digestive Masala (page 233)

1 tablespoon + 1 teaspoon olive oil

6 fresh curry leaves

¾ teaspoon salt, or to taste

½ teaspoon cumin seeds

2 black cardamom pods, slightly crushed open on one end

1 teaspoon maple syrup

½ teaspoon beet powder or 1 tablespoon fresh beet juice (for a rich red color)

⅛ teaspoon apple cider vinegar or fresh lime juice (optional)

1. In a medium saucepan, combine 1 cup water, the cranberries, tamarind pulp, masala, olive oil, curry leaves, salt, cumin seeds, and black cardamom. Bring to a boil over medium heat, then lower the heat, and simmer uncovered for 15 minutes, or until the tamarind and cranberries are soft. Set aside to cool.

2. Combine the cooked ingredients, the maple syrup, and beet powder in a blender, and blend until very smooth and creamy. Run the sauce through a fine-mesh strainer to separate any fibers (from the tamarind and black cardamom pods) and create an even creamier consistency. If the sauce turned out too thick, add a little water. Taste the sauce first without vinegar and then decide if it is sour enough for you (sometimes the less ripe tamarind is sour enough and will eliminate the need for vinegar).

3. Serve at room temperature. Store refrigerated in an airtight container for up to ten days.

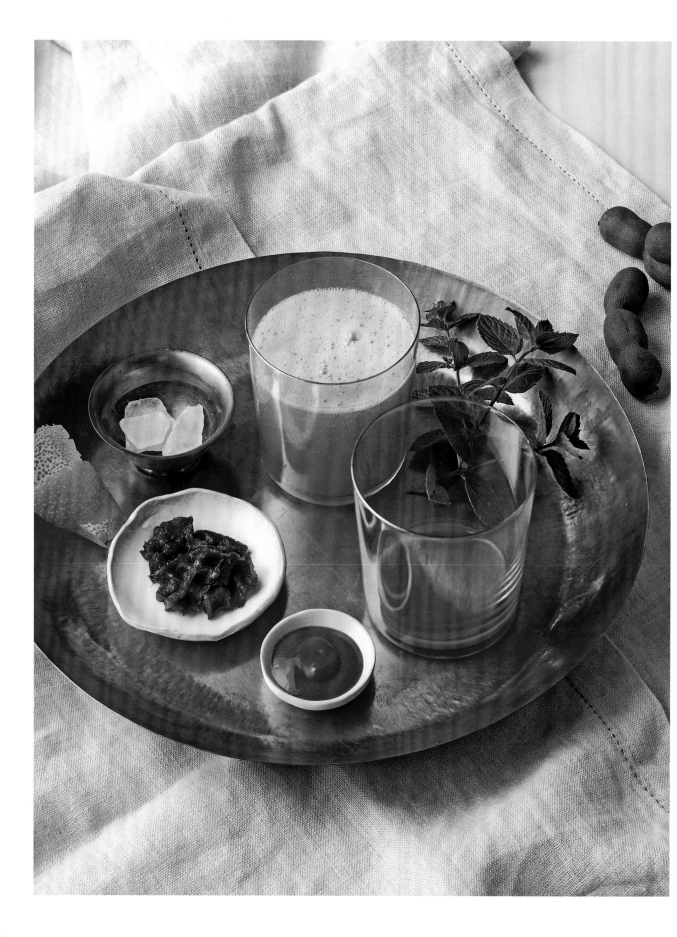

tamarind sherbet

MAKES concentrate for up to 9 servings • PREP: 10 minutes • COOK: 10 minutes • GF, DF • YEAR-ROUND

Tamarind sherbet is a favorite drink in many world cuisines, including Turkey, Iran, and Thailand. It's been cherished in India for thousands of years, and Ayurveda specifically mentions the sherbet in the category of *panaka*, or drinks. Edible camphor may seem like an unusual ingredient, but it is used in many Ayurvedic drinks and remedies. Here camphor not only contributes to the cooling effect of this beverage but it also clears congestion and tonifies the brain.

Tamarind Sherbet is another menu item from Divya's Kitchen. It is very rare for a restaurant chef to use time-consuming fresh tamarind, but I choose to because we could all benefit from its high mineral content and valuable traits. This drink is supremely refreshing and a very enjoyable way to improve your digestion and balance the three doshas. Drink it slightly chilled in the summer to relieve dehydration or warm in the cold season to boost your metabolism.

TAMARIND CONCENTRATE

½ cup raw cane sugar or shaved jaggery

¼ cup (2 ounces) sweet tamarind pulp
   (see Variation)

2 tablespoons grated fresh ginger

2 tablespoons chopped fresh mint
   (or 2 teaspoons dried mint)

4 cardamom pods

2-inch cinnamon stick

1 tablespoon dried rose petals

1 teaspoon orange zest

¼ cup fresh orange juice

2 tablespoons fresh lime juice

Pinhead amount of natural edible
   camphor crystal (optional)

To make the concentrate:

1. In a small saucepan, bring 2 cups water to a boil over medium-high heat. Add the sugar, tamarind, ginger, mint, cardamom, cinnamon, rose petals, and orange zest. Stir well, cover, lower the heat to low, and simmer for 10 minutes. Set aside uncovered and let it cool.

2. Remove the cinnamon and cardamom. In a blender, combine the cooked tamarind, orange juice, lime juice, and camphor. Blend until smooth, then strain through a fine-mesh strainer.

3. Store the concentrate in an airtight container in the refrigerator for up to five days.

To make 1 serving of the sherbet:

4. Pour ⅓ cup of the concentrate into a glass, and add 1 cup still or sparkling water. Stir and mix well. Enjoy with lunch or early dinner.

VARIATION: If you prefer to use fresh tamarind paste (see page 172), make the paste from 4 ounces of pods with their shells removed.

Opposite (counterclockwise): Tamarind Sherbet, edible camphor, tamarind pulp, tamarind paste

COCONUT

When I think of coconut trees, I reminisce about the tall palms along Miami Beach, Sunset Boulevard in Beverly Hills, and the dirt roads in Mayapur, India. When I lived in Mayapur (in Bengal), I was astonished to observe how sustainable the coconut is. The locals use all parts of the tree: they slice open young coconuts to drink the water and then scrape out the coconut meat and eat it right away. They recycle the husk to be used for sleeping mattresses: to do this, they chop and spread the husk onto the road so the passing cars loosen the fibers and then they leave the pieces to dry. The meat from mature coconuts is sliced or grated to make sweets, chutneys, curries; pressed into oil; or dehydrated. The villagers weave the palm leaves for cottage roofing or hand fans. Being highly nutritious and rich in fiber, good fats, vitamins, and minerals, coconut is the one plant that can help you survive on an uncharted and uninhabited island.

BOTANICAL NAME • *Cocos nucifera*
SANSKRIT NAME • *Narikela*

AYURVEDIC ATTRIBUTES

TASTE • sweet
QUALITIES • oily, heavy to digest, bulky
METABOLIC EFFECT • cooling
POST-DIGESTIVE EFFECT • sweet
DOSHA EFFECTS • pacifies Vata and Pitta, increases Kapha
HEALING BENEFITS • nourishes the hair

COMMON COCONUT PRODUCTS

COCONUT WATER

Slightly sweet, light to digest, Pitta pacifying, and deeply hydrating, coconut water is nature's best electrolyte drink. Enjoy coconut water during the hot hours of the day (not at night), when you need to

- relieve thirst or hydrate,
- cool down the heat in your body,
- stop hiccups,
- strengthen your bladder,
- eliminate kidney stones,
- alleviate burning urination,
- support your heart and reproductive system, and/or
- reduce a burning sensation on your skin (apply it topically).

COCONUT MEAT AND MILK

The meat from both young and mature coconut is sweet, cooling, and heavy to digest.

I make coconut milk by blending young coconut meat with water. It is helpful to deal with urinary disorders, hyperacidity, bleeding disorders, and to reduce flatulence.

Mature coconut meat is aphrodisiac and stimulates or increases menstrual flow. It also helps build the bulk tissues of the body.

COCONUT OIL

I use both unrefined (virgin) and refined coconut oil. The virgin oil is raw and heavier, with a noticeable smell and taste of coconut. I use it to cook under 375°F, in raw desserts, and for skin application. For higher temperature cooking, I use coconut oil that has been refined through a low heat steaming process, without the use of chemicals. This oil has less of a coconut aroma and taste and a higher smoke point; it is the preferred type for roasting or panfrying.

Applied externally, coconut oil is a renowned hair tonic. It nourishes and strengthens your hair, prevents or reverses hair loss, and also reduces heat in your head. If you decide to try it as a hair oil or hair lotion, apply enough to massage the scalp (there should be no dripping oil), and leave it for an hour or two, then wash it off with shampoo. Do not leave the coconut oil on your scalp overnight or apply during the cold season because the oil will congest your head.

Coconut oil is also antibacterial and antifungal when applied both internally and externally. Coconut oil counteracts dryness and burning sensations anywhere on your skin—dry patches on your cheeks or elbows, eczema, sunburns, stove or oven burns, nail fungus, and active hemorrhoids, and the burning sensation that comes after chopping fresh chiles.

In the last few decades, research has proven that coconut oil carries the good type of saturated fat that supplies balanced fatty lubrication for the brain.

SOURCING

- Coconut water, milk, meat, and oil have been staples in the diets of the Asian, Pacific, and other tropical island populations for generations. In cooler climates, you can purchase coconut products in grocery stores. I highly recommend making fresh milk from the meat of a young coconut over using canned coconut milk.

SEASON

- Because coconut is so cooling, summer is the best season to enjoy any of its forms. Drinking a glass of coconut water in the morning will help your body remain cool and tolerant of the day's heat.

DIGESTIBILITY

- Coconut in any form, except for coconut water, is heavy to digest. It calls for strong *agni*.
- If your *agni* fluctuates or you experience symptoms of Kapha imbalance, such as weight gain, congestion, bronchitis, or poor circulation, then avoid coconut products until you restore your balance.
- If you happen to get indigestion from eating too much coconut meat, try eating a teaspoon of coconut palm sugar as an antidote.

COOKING TIPS

- Use pungent spices, such as ginger and chile, to cut through the heaviness of coconut in any of its forms.

coconut chutney

MAKES about 2 cups ● PREP: 5 minutes ●
COOK: 3 minutes ● GF, DF ● SUMMER ●
Photograph on page 95

Coconut chutney is a favorite condiment in South India because of its cooling and nourishing properties. I learned this recipe from Vaidya Mishra, who recommended it for growing beautiful hair. If I told you that eating a delicious sauce regularly would make your hair thick and shiny, would you dare to try it?

2 tablespoons yellow split mung dal

1 cup diced, peeled mature fresh coconut (4½ ounces) or ¾ cup fine shredded dried coconut

1 tablespoon fresh lime juice

2 teaspoons olive oil

6 fresh curry leaves (optional)

½ teaspoon Protein Digestive Masala (page 233)

½ teaspoon salt, or to taste

FOR VATA OR PITTA BALANCING: Enjoy as is.

FOR KAPHA BALANCING: Add 1 seeded green Indian or Thai chile with the ingredients in Step 2.

1. In a small skillet, dry-toast the mung over medium-low heat until it turns a light brown color, about 3 minutes. Make sure to shake it frequently because mung can burn quickly. Transfer to a spice grinder and let it cool, then grind to a powder.

2. In a blender, combine 1 cup water with the ground mung, coconut, lime juice, olive oil, curry leaves, masala, and salt. Blend to a medium-thick, smooth paste (add more water if your chutney is too thick). Serve immediately or refrigerate in an airtight container for up to two days.

coconut-lavender shake

SERVES 5 to 6 ● PREP: 15 minutes (with already made Lavender Syrup) ● GF, DF ● SUMMER

I created this recipe for Divya's Kitchen during one very hot summer in New York City. I wanted to offer a cooling and hydrating beverage that also prevented skin dryness after sun exposure.

Each glass of Coconut-Lavender Shake is a piece of art—the semi-frozen cube of Lavender Syrup melts gradually, swirling hues of light purple in the snow-white coconut milk.

Enjoy this drink when you need something refreshing, relaxing, and uplifting. Lavender is also known to reduce feelings of agitation and insecurity. Well then, bring it on and serve it worldwide!

5 ounces fresh coconut meat (from 1 young coconut), chopped (1 cup)

⅓ cup fresh lime juice

¼ cup light colored raw cane sugar

1 piece (1 tablespoon) Lavender Syrup (recipe follows), semi-frozen

GARNISH

Fresh or dried lavender flowers

1. In a blender, combine 4 cups water with the coconut meat, lime juice, and sugar, and blend until very smooth and creamy. Strain through a fine-mesh strainer.

2. Whisk in 2½ cups more water, transfer to a pitcher, and refrigerate.

3. To serve: Fill a glass with the sweetened coconut milk, add the Lavender Syrup, and garnish with a sprinkle of lavender flowers. Serve with a straw that can also be used as a stirrer.

Lavender Syrup

MAKES ½ cup ● PREP: 30 minutes ●
COOK: 2 minutes ● FREEZE: 2 hours ●
GF, DF ● SUMMER

¼ cup raw cane sugar

3 tablespoons blueberries

2½ teaspoons dried lavender flowers

1. In a small saucepan, bring ½ cup water to a boil over medium-high heat, and stir in the sugar, blueberries, and lavender. Lower the heat, and simmer uncovered for 1 minute to dissolve the sugar.

2. Remove from the heat, cover, and let the lavender steep in the syrup for 20 minutes.

3. Strain through a fine-mesh strainer. Your syrup will have a beautiful deep purple color. Let it cool to room temperature, then pour it into ice cube trays and freeze for at least 2 hours. This syrup will not turn into ice completely; rather, it will have a semi-frozen texture.

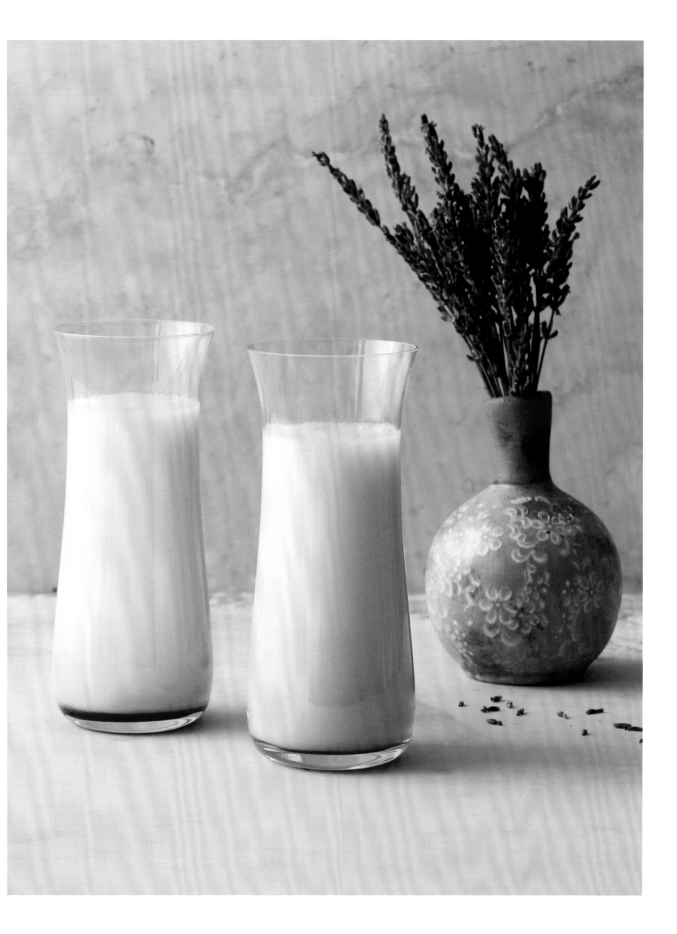

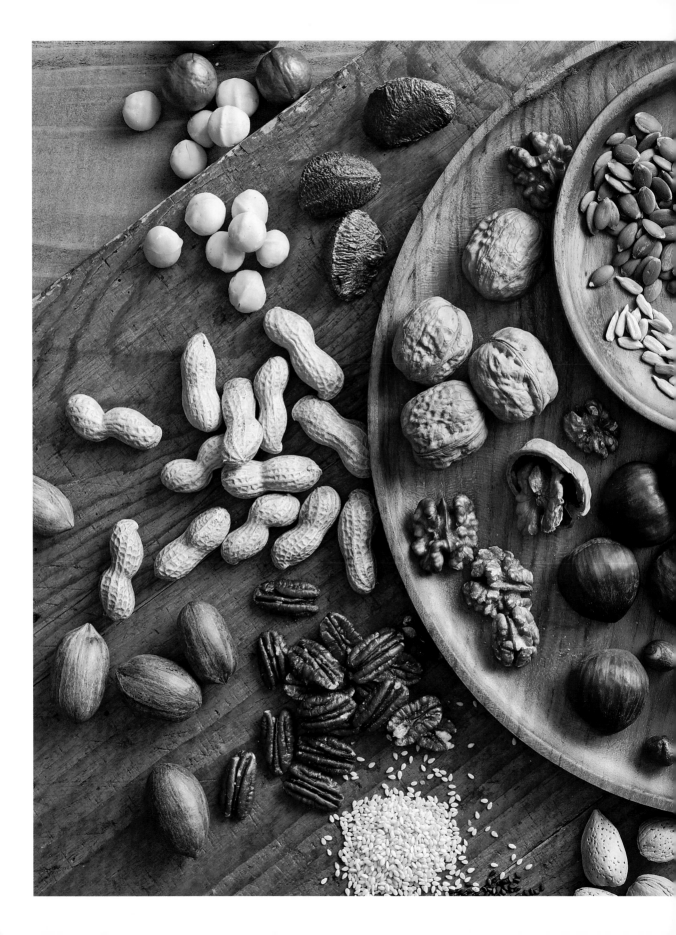

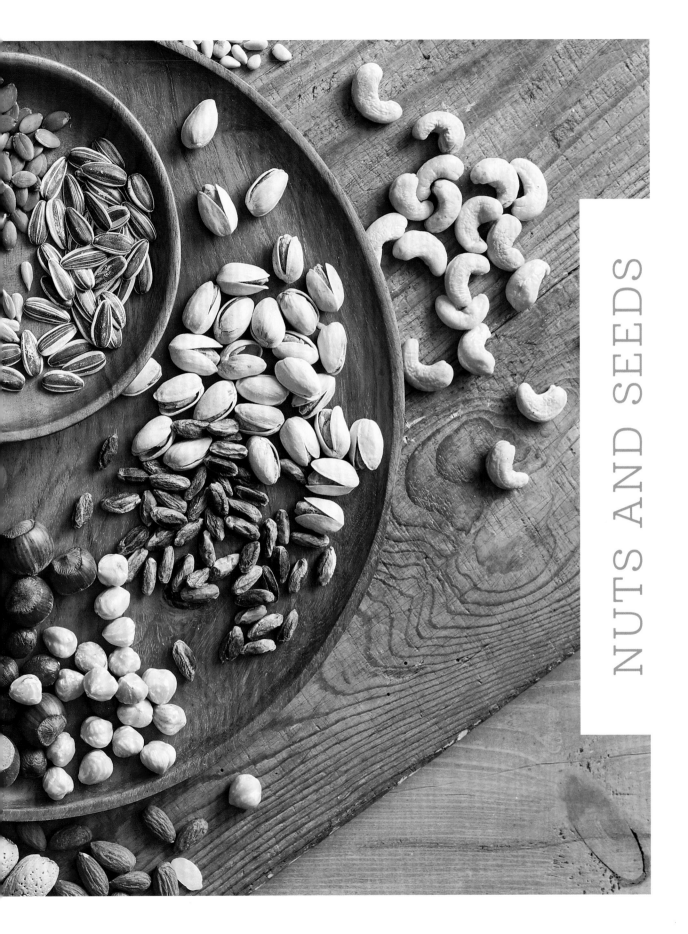

NUTS AND SEEDS

NUTS AND SEEDS

examples:

almonds

cashews

walnuts

pecans

hazelnuts

pistachios

macadamias

chestnuts

peanuts

pine nuts

Brazil nuts

———

sesame

sunflower

pumpkin

hemp

flax

chia

One childhood memory I recreate whenever I visit my father at his house in the mountains of Bulgaria is roaming in the woods and cracking young hazelnuts and walnuts from the trees that grow wild in that area. As a child, I used to imagine that I was on a nut-hunting expedition, seizing my found treasure from the tree branches before the squirrels claimed their nut prize. I felt so accomplished when I foraged a few handfuls of young nuts in their green shells, then cracked them open and marveled at the deliciousness of their tender, sweet, and supple kernels. Aside from storing walnuts for the winter, my grandmother would make a preserve with baby green walnuts, each jar seasoned with a sprig of rose geranium. I dream about tasting that special preserve once again.

Nuts are technically shell fruits, and the ancient Ayurvedic texts also classify them in the fruit category. Nuts are rich in good fats, proteins, vitamin E, calcium, magnesium, and potassium. Their biochemical effect surpasses the support that their nutrients provide our physiology. Ayurveda incorporates nuts as a restorative food—that which revives strength, builds body mass, and enhances the cognitive functions of the mind, including memory. Almonds are listed as the best among nuts.

SOURCING

- Buy only raw nuts from a recent harvest, and organic whenever possible. Although cracking the shells of nuts is rather labor intensive, nuts in their protective shell have the longest shelf life.
- Store shelled nuts in airtight containers, in a dark and dry place, preferably refrigerated, to reduce chances of rancidity. Nuts go rancid when their oils oxidize, which creates quite a toxic substance in the body. If your nuts have a sharp acidic smell and an unpleasant sour taste, discard them.

SEASON

- Different nuts mature during various times of the year. The best seasons to eat more nuts are the late fall and winter, when our body needs heavier foods, rich in healthy fats and protein.

DIGESTIBILITY

- Nuts are heavy to digest; therefore it is best to eat them in small amounts. In general, all tree nuts help balance Vata but increase Pitta and Kapha. Soaking the nuts (see chart on page 184) makes them much easier to digest, more alkalinizing, and balancing for all doshas.
- Lightly roasting the nuts also makes them more digestible, but the key is to roast them just before serving and to eat them all that day to minimize the chances of rancidity.
- Nut butters are naturally quite acidic and much harder to digest than whole nuts; they tend to be a clogging food.

COOKING TIPS

- To roast nuts, spread them dry on a baking sheet, and roast them at 300°F for 5 to 10 minutes, until they have a light tan color. Nuts that have been roasted too long or at a high temperature (as seen in roasted nuts with a dark color) carry the risk of damaged oils, making them less desirable for our health.
- You can also toast nuts over low heat in a dry skillet or coated with a little bit of oil and spices such as ginger, chiles, and curry leaves.

WALNUTS

BOTANICAL NAME ● *Juglans regia*

SANSKRIT NAME ● *Akshotakah*

Walnuts are of sweet taste, heavy to digest, Vata balancing, and have a heating metabolic effect. Ayurveda uses them to calm the nerves, increase appetite, and enhance stamina. Application of walnut oil on the skin promotes a good complexion and reduces inflammation and pain. The bark powder of the walnut tree is used as a tooth powder, as it makes the gums strong.

PECANS

BOTANICAL NAME ● *Carya illinoensis*

SANSKRIT NAME ● Unknown

A relative of walnuts, pecans are a native American crop. They are astringent and slightly sweet in taste, oily, heavy to digest, and have a heating metabolic effect. They are rich in good fats, protein, and vitamin B_6, and they help lower cholesterol.

PISTACHIOS

BOTANICAL NAME ● *Pistacia vera*

SANSKRIT NAME ● Unknown

The pleasantly green pistachios are of sweet taste, oily, energizing, and have a heating metabolic effect. They are a good source of zinc and phosphorus. The Sicilian variety of pistachios are renowned for their exceptionally bright green color.

PINE NUTS

BOTANICAL NAME ● *Pinus pinea* and others

SANSKRIT NAME ● Unknown

Technically seeds, pine nuts are perhaps most known for their use in Italian cuisine, especially in pesto. They are of astringent and sweet tastes and have a heating metabolic effect. Compared to all other nuts, pine nuts are the easiest to digest. They are very nutritive, enhance stamina, and stimulate energy.

CONTINUED ON PAGE 193

nut or seed milk

MAKES about 3 cups ● **SOAK:** varies (see below) ● **PREP:** about 5 minutes ● **GF, DF** ● **YEAR-ROUND**

Here is a base recipe for making a staple fresh nut or seed milk, which you can use as a substitute for dairy milk or even buttermilk when you add a bit of lime juice (especially in baking). Fresh plant milk is always more wholesome, nourishing, and delicious than its store-bought counterpart, which often comes with chemical preservatives. Try making it at least once.

Use the proportions below, and follow these steps to make your plant milk:

1. Rinse and drain the nuts or seeds, then soak for the recommended duration.

2. Drain and rinse.

3. Blend with the recommended amount of filtered or spring water plus a pinch of salt.

4. Strain through a nut milk bag, layered cheesecloth, or fine-mesh strainer (with the exception of cashews). Refrigerate or freeze the remaining pulp in an airtight container for another use (see Note).

5. Store the milk in a jar, bottle, or other air-tight container, and refrigerate for up to three days. Shake well before using.

NOTE: The leftover pulp from making fresh nut or seed milk has many uses—try it in baked goods, raw desserts, or as a thickener and added source of protein in soups and smoothies.

1 cup raw nuts or seeds	Soak in 3 cups of water for:	Blend with . . . water	Strain
Almonds	8 hours	3 cups	Yes
Cashews	8 hours	3½ cups	No
Hazelnuts	6 hours	3 cups	Yes
Walnuts	6 hours	3 cups	Yes
Sunflower Seeds	4 hours	3 cups	Yes
Pumpkin Seeds	4 hours	3 cups	Yes

cashew gravy

MAKES 1½ cups ● SOAK: 8 hours or overnight ● PREP: 5 minutes ● COOK: about 5 minutes ● GF, DF ●
FALL-WINTER ● Photograph on page 115

What comes to mind when you hear the word *gravy*? A roast? Mashed potatoes? Biscuits? Growing up in Bulgaria, gravy was not really in my family's meal repertoire. When I moved to the US, where gravy is deeply embedded in the culinary culture—and not just in the meat-eating culture—I came to appreciate how gravy adds moisture and flavor to drier foods. I created this recipe years ago for a festive vegetarian meal during the winter holidays. You can't have Thanksgiving without gravy, but you can have gravy without meat!

This flavorful, multiuse gravy is especially suitable during the cold season. Its moist creaminess will complement steamed, roasted, or stuffed vegetables, pasta, biscuits, and more. Serve it with Stuffed Cabbage Rolls (page 113), Sesame Crackers (page 68), Gluten-Free Paratha Flatbread (page 56), or Braised Purple Cabbage (page 117).

½ cup cashews, soaked in water for at least 8 hours or overnight, rinsed, and drained

1 tablespoon arrowroot powder

1 tablespoon nutritional yeast

1¼ teaspoons salt, or to taste

Tiny pinch of asafoetida

1 teaspoon Za'atar (page 234)

¼ teaspoon freshly ground black pepper

1. In a blender, blend the cashews with 1 cup water until it has reached a smooth, creamy consistency.

2. Add another 1 cup water, the arrowroot, nutritional yeast, salt, and asafoetida. Briefly blend again to mix the ingredients.

3. Transfer the mixture to a 1½-quart saucepan and bring to a simmer over medium-low heat. Whisk frequently to prevent lumps as the sauce thickens. Once the gravy starts bubbling, turn off the heat, and whisk in the Za'atar and pepper. The consistency of this gravy is not too runny and not too thick—it should slowly flow from a spoon. Of course, you can adjust the thickness to your liking by adding or reducing the water.

4. Serve hot or warm. Store covered in the refrigerator for up to three days.

cashew sour cream

MAKES about 1 cup ● SOAK: 8 hours or overnight ● PREP: 5 minutes ● GF, DF ● YEAR-ROUND ● Photograph on page 116

This is a great substitute for common sour cream—it has the creaminess and tanginess of its dairy counterpart, but it is much lighter to digest. At Divya's Kitchen, we use it to garnish avocado toast, savory waffles, pancakes, and more.

¾ cup cashews, soaked in water for at least 8 hours or overnight, rinsed, and drained

1 tablespoon fresh lime juice

¼ teaspoon salt

1. Combine the cashews, ⅓ cup water, the lime juice, and salt in a blender, and blend to a smooth and creamy consistency. Adjust the water and seasonings to your liking.

2. Store refrigerated for up to five days.

VARIATIONS: Create a new flavor or color by blending in any combination of the following:

¼ teaspoon toasted ground cumin

¼ teaspoon freshly ground black pepper

2 tablespoons chopped fresh parsley or cilantro leaves

1 green Indian or Thai chile

1 tablespoon fresh beet juice

cashew vanilla cream

MAKES about 1 cup ● SOAK: 8 hours or overnight ● PREP: 5 minutes ● GF, DF ● YEAR-ROUND ● Photograph on page 190

In the West, we love topping our fruit salad, pie, cobbler, pancakes, or waffles with whipped cream, but Ayurveda considers the combination of dairy with these dishes to upset digestion. Cashew Vanilla Cream is a delicious dairy-free alternative that provides equal satisfaction.

¾ cup cashews, soaked in water for at least 8 hours or overnight, rinsed, and drained

2½ tablespoons raw cane sugar or maple syrup

1 teaspoon fresh lime juice

½ teaspoon vanilla extract

¼ teaspoon ground cardamom

Tiny pinch of salt

1. Combine the cashews, ¼ cup water, the cane sugar, lime juice, vanilla, cardamom, and salt in a blender, and blend to a smooth and creamy consistency. Adjust the water and seasonings to your liking.

2. Store refrigerated for up to five days.

pistachio fudge

MAKES: about thirty 1-inch squares ● **PREP**: 10 minutes ● **COOK**: 50 minutes ● **CHILL**: 2 hours ● **GF, DF** ● **YEAR-ROUND**

When you hear *fudge*, you may think *chocolate*, but it doesn't have to be this way. The concept of fudge—creamy candy cooked down in milk—can be applied in a variety of ways, such as the traditional Indian fudge desserts burfi and sandesh. This recipe resembles a much lighter version of pistachio burfi—I use almond milk instead of dairy and do not add any fat because the nuts are already quite fatty.

Cooking down the ground nuts to a fudge-like consistency takes time and patience, but the reward is that this sweet lasts for a while when refrigerated. You can make it in advance and keep it as a nice treat for unexpected guests or when you can't ignore your sweet tooth. Because it stores well, travels well, looks beautiful, and tastes sublime, this dessert is a favorite on Divya's Kitchen dining and catering menus.

There is something heavenly about Pistachio Fudge—its sweetness and nutty flavor will take you into a dreamy state. The brown-green color, chewy stickiness, and the way it melts in the mouth—this all amounts to a healthy enjoyment you deserve. Unleash your artistry when you shape the fudge. It is pliable enough to cut into squares or rectangles, roll into balls, or press into decorative molds.

2 cups (255 grams) raw shelled pistachios
1½ cups almond milk (see page 184)
⅔ cup (170 grams) raw cane sugar
¾ teaspoon ground cardamom
½ teaspoon vanilla extract

GARNISH

2 tablespoons finely ground pistachios (the Sicilian variety are of the brightest green color)

FOR VATA OR PITTA BALANCING: Enjoy as is.

FOR KAPHA BALANCING: This would be a bit heavy for you. Slowly savor a tiny piece.

1. Place the pistachios in a food processor, and grind them until they turn into a fine but not pasty meal. The consistency should be like a fine almond meal.

2. In a 10- to 12-inch skillet, combine the ground pistachios, almond milk, sugar, cardamom, and vanilla. Bring to a gentle simmer over medium-low heat. Turn down the heat to the lowest setting and continue to simmer, stirring frequently with a wooden spatula. The liquid will gradually evaporate, and the mixture will thicken to a sticky, fudge-like consistency; the thicker it gets, the more you need to stir to prevent burning and clumping. Cooking is complete when the mixture starts to form a single, thick mass, pulls away from the bottom of the pan, and the spatula leaves a clear passage on the bottom of the pan when you run it across. This will take about 40 minutes.

3. Transfer the fudge onto a cookie sheet layered with parchment paper. Spread it out, pat with a spatula, and mold the hot sticky mixture into a smooth cake, ½ inch thick. Place a piece of parchment paper on top of the fudge, and run a rolling pin over it with very little pressure, just enough to smooth the top surface while keeping the shape of the fudge cake.

4. Leave the fudge covered with the parchment paper, and refrigerate for at least 2 hours or overnight.

5. Cut the fudge into 1-inch squares or your desired shape (I recommend bite-size pieces). Keep refrigerated in an airtight container for up to two weeks. Bring to room temperature before serving, and just before plating, dust the fudge pieces with ground pistachios.

VARIATION: Replace the pistachios with almonds, hazelnuts, walnuts, or a combination of these.

the best cooking fats

- Cultured ghee is best among animal fats (saturated fat)—tridoshic; good to use all year round

- Sesame oil is best among seed oils (polyunsaturated fat)—balancing for Vata and Kapha; use occasionally in cold weather

- Olive oil is best among seed/fruit oils (high-quality extra virgin; monounsaturated fat)—tridoshic; good to use all year round

- Coconut oil is best among fruit oils (raw or nonchemically refined; saturated fat)—balancing for Vata and Pitta; good to use in hot weather

- Seeds are largely used to produce vegetable oils, such as canola (from rapeseed), soy, sunflower, sesame, safflower, pumpkin, mustard, corn, and grapeseed. However, in their unrefined state, these polyunsaturated oils don't live up to the average consumer's needs, so manufacturers hydrogenate them to increase their shelf life and smoke point and neutralize their flavor. The regular consumption of hydrogenated polyunsaturated fats has been linked to heart disease and an increase of bad cholesterol. It is best to avoid them for cooking (except for sesame oil). Unfortunately, most restaurants cook exclusively with hydrogenated oils because they are cheap and have a neutral flavor. Divya's Kitchen is a rare exception—we only use the four best cooking fats mentioned above.

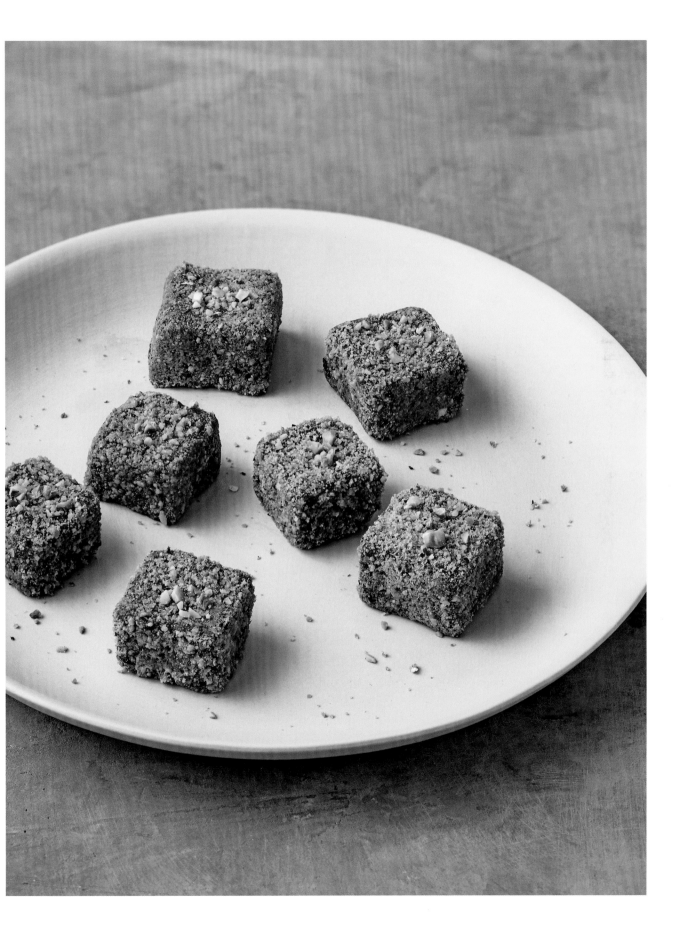

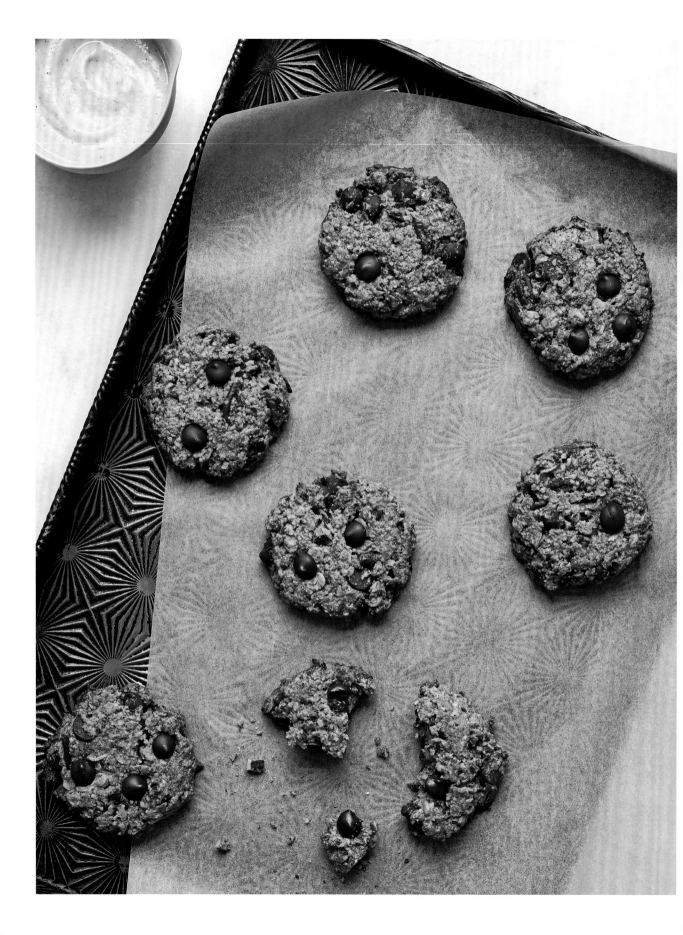

pecan chocolate chip cookies

MAKES nine 3-inch cookies ● **PREP:** 20 minutes ● **BAKE:** 40 minutes ● **GF, DF** ● **FALL-WINTER**

These are cookies of substance—they almost feel like a protein snack bar: rich in protein and fiber, very filling, and, most important, addictive. It's hard to believe that a cookie so delicious is gluten free, vegan, and sweetened without sugar. I think that among the hundreds of chocolate chip cookie recipes in the world, this version stands proudly on the health awards podium.

We serve them at Divya's Kitchen, and I've included the recipe in this book because our guests repeatedly ask me for it. Enjoy them freshly baked, with a dollop of Cashew Vanilla Cream (page 186) and a cup of tea.

1¾ cups (200 grams) pecan halves

¼ cup melted coconut oil or ghee, plus more for greasing

2 cups (186 grams) rolled oats, divided

¼ cup + 2 tablespoons (44 grams) sorghum flour

¼ cup + 1 tablespoon (44 grams) amaranth flour

1 teaspoon Sweet Masala #2 (page 234)

½ teaspoon ground cinnamon

½ teaspoon baking soda

¼ teaspoon salt

½ cup maple syrup (room temperature or warmed)

2 tablespoons almond milk (see page 184)

2 tablespoons fresh lime juice

1 teaspoon vanilla extract

⅓ cup pitted dates (60 grams), finely chopped

½ cup (90 grams) mini chocolate chips (ideally semisweet, soy free)

1. Preheat the oven to 300°F. Line a half-size sheet pan with a silicone mat or piece of parchment paper.

2. Spread the pecans on the pan, and roast them for 10 minutes, or until the nuts are crispy and slightly darker; set them aside to cool. Coarsely chop ¾ cup of the pecans.

3. Increase the oven temperature to 350°F. Grease the lining of the same sheet pan with coconut oil.

4. In a food processor, grind the 1 cup unchopped toasted pecans and 1 cup of the oats to a coarse meal. Transfer to a large bowl, and fold in the remaining pecans, the rolled oats, sorghum and amaranth flours, masala, cinnamon, baking soda, and salt. Mix well.

5. In a medium bowl, whisk together the maple syrup, coconut oil, almond milk, lime juice, and vanilla. Fold in the chopped dates and the chocolate chips.

6. Add the wet ingredients to the dry mixture, and combine well to make a coarse, sticky batter.

7. Using your wet hands or a spoon, shape the cookie batter into nine equal portions, and place them 1 inch apart from each other on the sheet pan. You can also make them smaller, according to your preferred size.

8. Bake for 30 minutes (or less for smaller-size cookies), or until the cookies are crusty and golden on the outside and cooked on the inside. Keep in mind that the cookies will be soft as soon as you take them out of the oven but will firm up as they cool down.

9. Serve them warm or at room temperature.

care for dry skin

A lot of us experience dry skin, especially during the cold, windy months. Dryness can also occur from using chemical-based skin care products, including makeup. There are many natural ways to keep our face clean, moist, and wrinkle free. Here are some ideas.

You'll find cleanser recipes for oily skin on page 54 and for sensitive skin on page 93.

skin cleansing powder for dry skin

This powder offers a gentle exfoliation and a deep wash of the top layer of the facial skin. The almond meal's texture lends a soft scrubbing action, and its bit of fat balances the drying effects of the mung flour. Use it each morning and evening.

2 tablespoons fine almond meal
1 tablespoon whole mung flour (see Note)
1 teaspoon raw cane sugar
1 teaspoon dried lavender flowers (optional)

TO MAKE: Mix all the ingredients with a mortar and pestle. Store in a dry, airtight container, away from light (I keep it in the bathroom vanity).

TO USE: In your palm, add ½ teaspoon of the cleansing powder and enough warm water to make a thin but not runny paste. (If your skin is very dry, then use heavy cream or coconut milk instead of water.) Apply the paste all over your face, and gently massage into the skin for about 1 minute. Do not scrub. Rinse well with warm (not hot) water. Let your skin air-dry. Follow up with a toner and moisturizer of your choice.

probiotic mask for dry skin

This mask offers a deep cleaning of the pores and restores the friendly bacteria in your skin. Use it once or twice a week. Manjishtha is a famous Ayurvedic herb known to improve complexion and bind toxins in the liver, blood, and skin.

1 teaspoon whole mung flour or oat flour
¼ teaspoon manjishtha powder (optional)
About 1 teaspoon plain whole yogurt

TO MAKE: Mix the flour and manjishtha, and add enough plain yogurt to create a medium-thick paste.

TO USE: Apply the mask on your cleaned face, leave it for 10 minutes, and rinse off with warm water. Let your skin air-dry. Follow up with a toner and moisturizer of your choice.

NOTE: To make whole mung flour, use a spice grinder to grind 1 to 2 tablespoons of whole mung beans into a fine powder. You can also purchase it from Indian grocery stores (labeled as "Green Gram Flour").

CONTINUED FROM PAGE 183

SESAME SEEDS

BOTANICAL NAME • *Sesamum indicum*

SANSKRIT NAME • *Tila*

Ayurveda highly values sesame seeds because they have a slightly heating metabolic effect and are very balancing for Vata. Rich in calcium and iron, sesame seeds are one of the best ingredients to keep our bones, hair, and nails strong. Toasting sesame seeds before using them whole or grinding them into a paste (tahini) is important in order to make them more bioavailable.

SUNFLOWER SEEDS

BOTANICAL NAME • *Helianthus annuus*

SANSKRIT NAME • *Suryakanti*

Sunflower seeds are of sweet taste, heavy to digest (but lighter than nuts), have a cooling metabolic effect, and are tridoshic but most balancing for Vata. As a nurturing and building food, sunflower seeds are a good source of iron, calcium, phenolic antioxidants, and vitamin E, and they contain more protein than beef by volume.

Eat them in moderation, especially if your kidneys tend to form oxalate-type stones.

Nuts and seeds can be interchangeable in most recipes. I use sunflower seeds to make milk and dips for someone with nut allergies.

sunflower-herb dressing

MAKES about 2 cups • **PREP:** 10 minutes • **GF, DF** • **YEAR-ROUND**

I love how simple and versatile this dressing is. It goes well with any kind of lettuce salad and steamed vegetable, or you can serve it as a sauce for cooked grains, sautéed leafy greens, roasted vegetables, and more.

5 tablespoons olive oil

3 tablespoons fresh lime juice

⅔ cup roasted sunflower seeds (see Note on page 194)

1 teaspoon salt

½-inch piece fresh ginger, peeled and chopped

¼ cup chopped fresh basil leaves

2 tablespoons chopped fresh parsley leaves

Place all the ingredients in a blender, add 1 cup water, and blend until smooth. Store refrigerated in an airtight container for up to two days.

sunflower-beet hummus

MAKES about 1½ cups ● **SOAK:** 2 hours ● **PREP:** 15 minutes ● **COOK:** 10 minutes ● **GF, DF** ●
SUMMER-FALL-WINTER

This enchanting pink dip is a real crowd pleaser. We've served it on cucumber rings and crackers as finger food at multiple events, and it is also a popular appetizer at Divya's Kitchen. Hummus doesn't have to have a bean base. By substituting sunflower seeds for the traditional chickpea or another bean, I preserve the taste, texture, and protein content of the popular Middle Eastern dip and make it gentler on digestion.

For a colorful presentation, serve Sunflower-Beet Hummus (page 194) on a platter with Sesame Crackers (page 68), Roasted Carrot Tahini Sauce (page 148), thin celery or cucumber sticks, and microgreens; spread it on toast or wrap it in a tortilla.

1 small red beet, peeled and thinly sliced (about ¾ cup)

2 teaspoons olive oil

⅛ teaspoon asafoetida

½ cup sunflower seeds, soaked in water for 2 hours, rinsed, and drained

½ cup roasted sunflower seeds (see Note)

¼ cup tahini

3 tablespoons fresh orange juice

2 tablespoons fresh lime juice

1 teaspoon toasted ground cumin

1 teaspoon salt

½ teaspoon finely grated orange zest

GARNISHES

1 teaspoon dry-toasted kalonji seeds

2 teaspoons fresh lemon thyme leaves

1. Place the beets in a steamer basket in a small saucepan, and steam for 8 to 10 minutes, until soft. Set aside to cool and reserve the cooking water.

2. In the meantime, heat the olive oil and asafoetida in a small skillet over low heat until the asafoetida releases its aroma, about 5 seconds.

3. In a food processor, combine the beets, seasoned olive oil, raw and roasted sunflower seeds, tahini, orange and lime juice, cumin, salt, orange zest, and ½ cup of the beet steaming water, and process until smooth. Stop a few times and, using a rubber spatula, push down the ingredients that stick to the sides of the bowl. Transfer to a serving bowl, and garnish with toasted kalonji seeds and lemon thyme leaves.

4. Serve slightly chilled or at room temperature. Refrigerated in an airtight container, this dip will last up to three days.

NOTE: To roast the sunflower seeds: Preheat the oven (or a toaster oven) to 300°F. Spread the seeds on a small baking dish, and roast for about 5 minutes, until they are slightly golden. You can also toast the seeds in a pan on the stovetop over low heat. Be careful to not roast the seeds to a dark brown color—otherwise, your hummus will taste quite bitter.

Opposite (counterclockwise): Sunflower-Beet Hummus, Roasted Carrot-Tahini Sauce, Spelt-Sesame Crackers, Gluten-Free Sesame Crackers

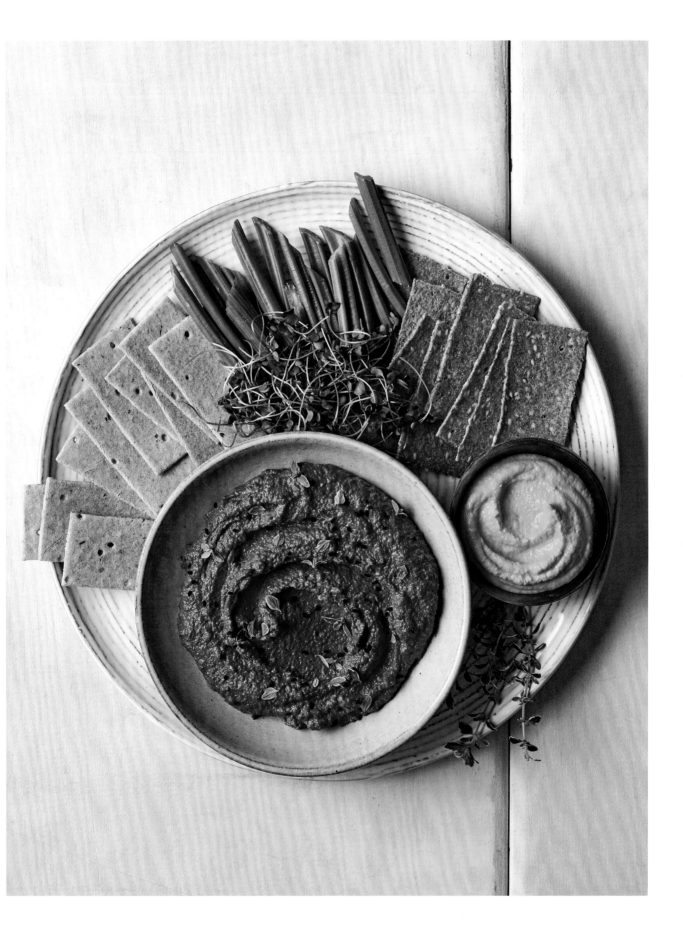

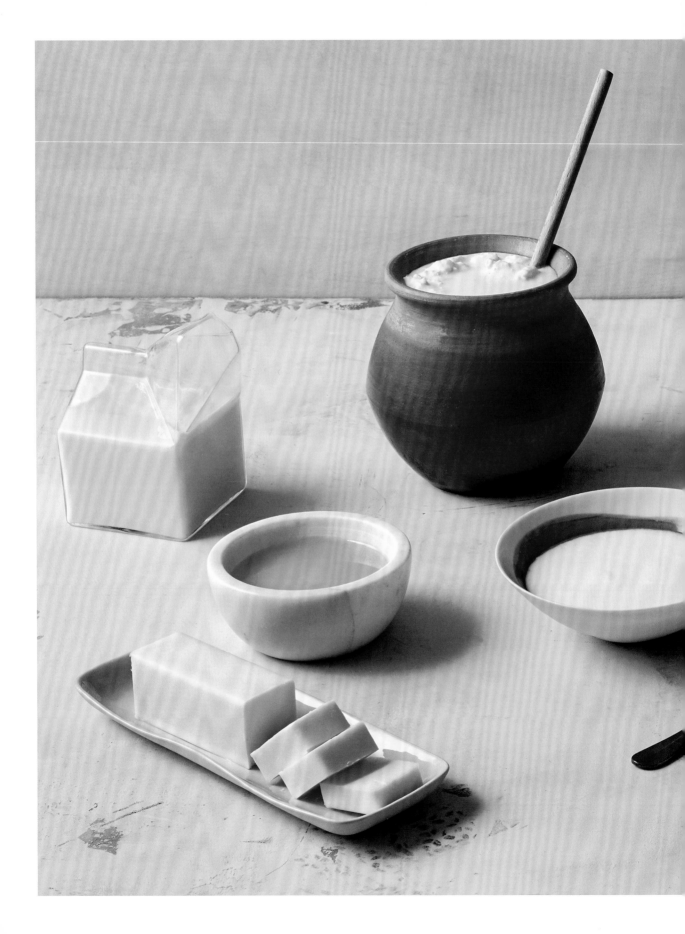

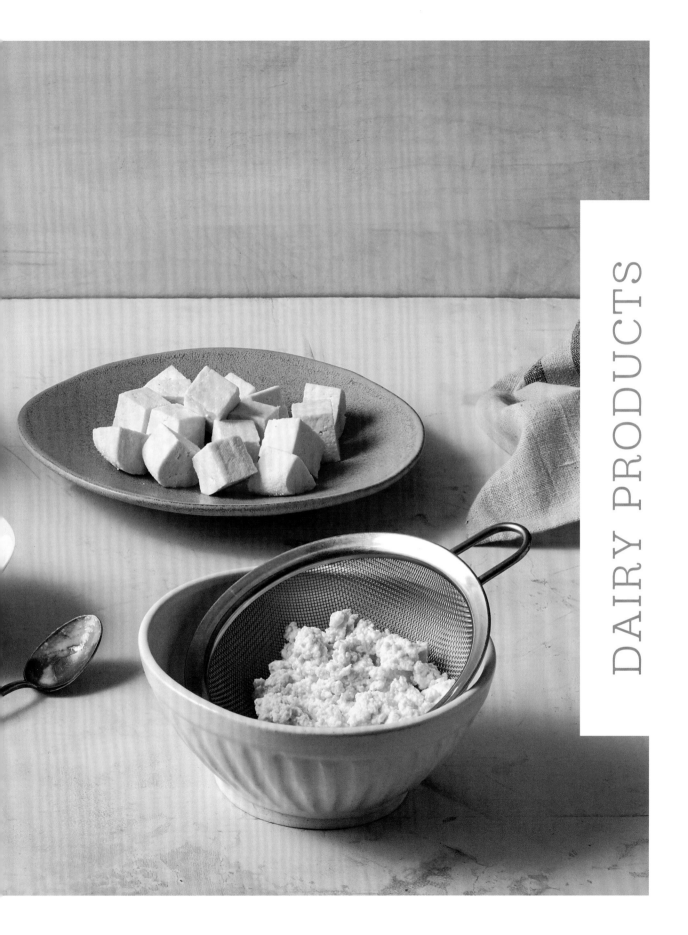

DAIRY PRODUCTS

My parents enjoy telling me the tale of how I drank milk directly from a cow's udder when I was about three years old, during a visit to my grandparents' dairy farm. I don't remember if I was hungry or if I wanted to imitate a calf, but the cow apparently remained very calm and treated me as her child.

It was in yoga class where I first heard about the Vedic concept of the cow being one of our mothers, so given my childhood experience, you can imagine how I immediately related.

Ever since I started practicing yoga and living a life of nonviolence as much as possible (that's one reason I became a vegetarian thirty-some years ago), I also began to consciously support cow care. Prentiss and I celebrated our wedding at the Gita Nagari Eco Farm in Pennsylvania, a place that takes care of about ninety cows for life, until they die naturally. Many of these cows come to the farm as slaughterhouse rescues. A couple of years ago, I visited Gita Nagari again, and I was astonished to learn that of their current nineteen milking cows, none of them had babies! They all gave milk without being induced, simply because they were happy and well cared for. Today, Gita Nagari continues to produce limited amounts of milk and cheese that is *ahimsa*, meaning that the milk comes from happy, grass-fed cows that

will never be killed. I believe this model of farming is the future of sustainable agriculture: it supports dairy production that can reverse the negative consequences of climate change, and it promotes affectionate relationships between humans and domestic animals.

Ayurveda and Vedic culture in general honor milk and milk products as some of the most sacred substances in life. The ancient textbooks emphatically state that milk is an appropriate food for all healthy individuals. In Vedic times, a person who was unable to digest milk was considered unhealthy and treated by physicians so that he or she could again consume milk. The ancient doctors were certain that the proper intake of milk would not lead to disease; in fact, they prescribed it therapeutically for many disorders.

Then why is it today that we have so many doubts about milk and its derivatives? Why do so many holistic health practitioners and doctors reject milk, as if it is poison? My Ayurveda studies helped me resolve the conflicting opinions about dairy, at least in terms of my own health.

For starters, not all milk is the same. Milk from unhappy, mistreated cows who live on unethical, conventional dairy farms is poison. Such milk is carrying the antibiotics and growth hormones given to the cows. Then it is subjected to more damage through the processes of pasteurization, homogenization, and fortification with artificial vitamins. That is poison.

However, there is nectar on the other side of the field. Ayurveda considers dairy-based nectar to be the milk that comes from well-cared for cows who happily graze in the fields and live without the fear of being slaughtered. Such milk and farms are rare, but they exist all over the world and gradually set a new model for sustainable and ethical farming.

In *What to Eat for How You Feel*, I address modern issues with dairy quality and consumption in a chapter called "The Dairy Question." Here is a brief summary.

SOURCING

- The best quality milk (and dairy products) is raw, organic, A2, whole, and from grass-fed cows. There are many yoga, Amish, and other family farms that provide this quality of milk all over the US. The next best quality, which you can buy in health food stores, is pasteurized but non-homogenized—still look for organic, A2, grass-fed, and ideally in a glass bottle.

- Ayurveda considers cow's milk to be the most suitable type of milk for human consumption (that is what I use in my recipes); however, it also outlines the properties of milk from elephants and even humans! Many people prefer goat's milk over cow's milk because it has a lighter consistency that makes it more digestible for them. That is fine; just keep in mind that goat's milk is of astringent taste (cow's is sweet), can imbalance Vata (cow's is tridoshic, more or less), and is best suited for mitigating Pitta and Kapha doshas.

SEASON

- Milk and milk products, such as yogurt, butter, buttermilk, and cheese have very different attributes and healing benefits; therefore it is important to adjust their consumption with the changes of seasons. In general, the following holds true:

- Milk is suitable in all seasons.
- Yogurt is best in the winter and the rainy season (in tropical regions).
- Butter in small quantity is best in the winter.
- Buttermilk works in all seasons.
- Ghee is good for cooking every day (bigger amounts in the fall and winter, less in the spring and summer).

DIGESTIBILITY

- Most people who react to dairy either consume it in a state of unwholesome quality, in the wrong way, or mix it with incompatible foods that cause a digestive reaction (see Ayurvedic Food Compatibility Chart, page 244). These are the common digestive mistakes we make when consuming milk and milk products.

Dairy Product	Improperly consumed when
Milk, heavy cream	cold, without spices, mixed with incompatible foods
Yogurt	cold, drained for thicker consistency (e.g., Greek yogurt), cooked (exception with baked goods), eaten at night, mixed with incompatible foods
Butter	cold, eating too much of it
Buttermilk	cold, without spices, cooked, drank at night
Cheese	cold, without spices, mixed with incompatible foods
Ghee	cold

- Cold dairy, even of the best quality, can turn into a clogging and unbalancing food. If you want to improve your relationship with dairy and benefit from its tremendous healing properties, try to shift your habits to use the best quality, consume it properly, and follow the compatibility guidelines. Despite all your best efforts, dairy might not be a wholesome food for your body right now—whether it is due to a genetic allergy predisposition, an intolerance developed over time, or an emotional aversion. If dairy does not sit well with you, don't force it on yourself.

COOKING TIPS

- Boiling: always bring milk to a boil over low heat—this will preserve its micronutrients.
- Avoid freezing and then reheating pasteurized milk because it becomes harder to digest (even if you drink it hot). Reheated frozen milk works best for someone with a very high Pitta imbalance (e.g., hot flashes, a burning sensation in the stomach, or high acidity).
- Don't microwave milk (or any food!)—this will kill all of the micronutrients that make milk healthy.
- Do not make milk from milk powder. Most milk powders are overly processed and include added chemicals.

DRINK HOT SPICED MILK WHEN YOU NEED TO (THIS IS FOR ANIMAL MILK ONLY, NOT OTHER MILK PRODUCTS)

- calm down and de-stress,
- gain physical and psychological strength,
- provide quick deep nourishment to your body (build *ojas*),
- gain weight after a depleting illness,
- improve your hormonal and cognitive functions,
- enhance your immune system,
- increase libido, and/or
- balance your Vata and Pitta.

FRESH CHEESE

I grew up eating cheese. From sweet, soft, and unfermented to briefly aged feta to hard-core cheddar—bread and cheese was the fastest way for me to fuel my body and go back to play with my friends. Years later, as I healed from my autoimmune disorder, I had to give up all aged cheeses. Sadly, I could not digest them, and they perpetuated my high acidity and chronic inflammation. Being healthy again, today I still stick to fresh cheeses only for two reasons: I love them and most of the rennet in aged cheeses is not vegetarian friendly.

AYURVEDIC ATTRIBUTES

TASTE ● sweet or slightly sour

QUALITIES ● heavy to digest, fatty, oily

METABOLIC EFFECT ● slightly heating

POST-DIGESTIVE EFFECT ● sweet or sour

DOSHA EFFECTS ● balances Vata and Pitta, increases Kapha

HEALING BENEFITS ● builds body mass, strengthens bones and muscles

COMMON TYPES OF FRESH CHEESE AVAILABLE TODAY

- white mozzarella
- cottage cheese
- goat's cheese
- ricotta
- farmer cheese
- paneer cheese

SOURCING

- In India, the fresh pressed cheese is called paneer, and the unpressed curds are called chenna. In the West, we seem to label both cheese textures as paneer.
- It is best to make fresh cheese at home. Indian grocery stores sell it frozen, but I never buy it because of its questionable milk source, lack of freshness, and very rubbery texture.

SEASON

- Especially if you're a vegetarian, fresh cheese can be your main source of animal protein in every season. Otherwise, it is better to eat it more frequently in the fall and winter, while slightly reducing your intake of it in the summer and much more in the spring.

DIGESTIBILITY

- The fresher the cheese, the easier it is to digest. And even then, it remains a heavy food; that's why it is important to prepare it with pungent spices, such as cardamom (black or green), black pepper, chiles, fenugreek, and ginger.
- Eat it at lunchtime, when *agni* is strongest.
- Favor cow's or goat's milk cheeses. Sheep's dairy aggravates the three doshas, and buffalo dairy is too heavy (recommended only for sleeplessness and excessive hunger pangs).

COOKING TIPS

- Use crumbled paneer cheese as a replacement for crumbled tofu.
- Blend unpressed paneer cheese with a little water and salt to make homemade cream cheese.
- Blend unpressed paneer cheese with a little water, powdered raw sugar, ground cardamom, orange zest, and vanilla to create a delectable frosting for cakes or muffins.
- Sear paneer cheese cubes with ghee in a pan, or bake them with ghee in the oven.
- If your cheese is hard, soak it in boiling hot water for about 30 minutes, or until it becomes soft and succulent.

EAT FRESH CHEESE WHEN YOU WANT TO

- add animal protein to your diet,
- gain weight,
- build muscle, and/or
- enrich your diet with calcium, vitamin B_{12}, and omega-3 fatty acids.

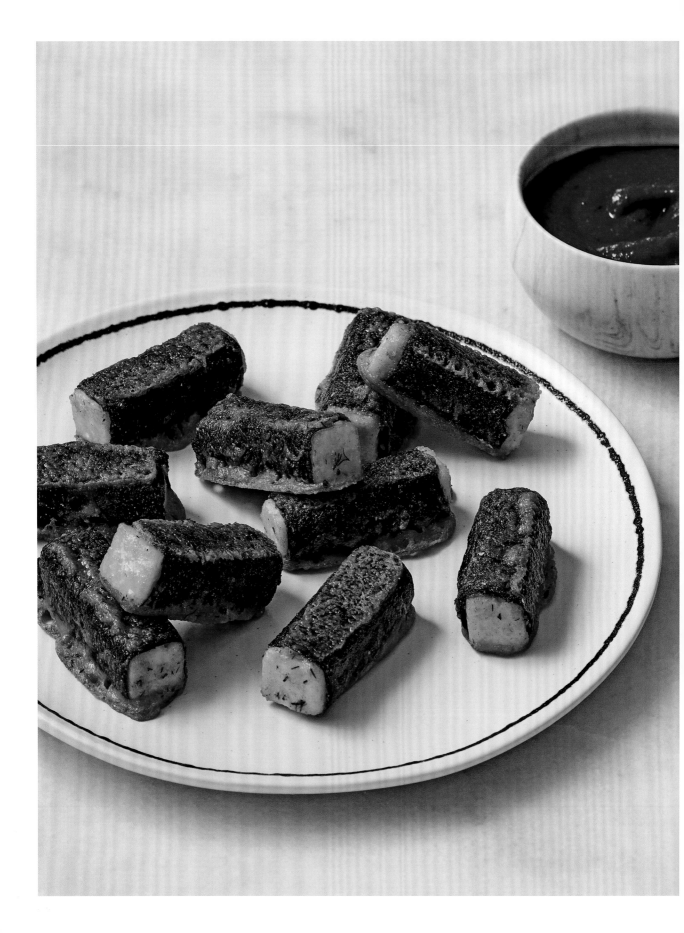

nori-cheese sticks

MAKES 8 sticks ● **PREP:** 20 minutes (with already made paneer cheese) ● **COOK:** about 10 minutes ●
GF ● **FALL-WINTER**

My friend and former cooking class instructor at Bhagavat Life Andriy Egorovets taught me this recipe many years ago. He called it "fish sticks" because of the white meaty texture of the cheese, the sea taste of the nori, and the golden-crusted batter that encompasses the whole morsel. The spongy cheese provides fullness, and that crispy and fatty crunch you love about eating deep-fried cheese sticks is certainly there. I immediately fell in love with them.

If it's more practical for you, prepare the cheese, the nori, and the batter ahead of time and keep them refrigerated. Start panfrying the cheese sticks right before mealtime, and keep them in a warm oven until serving. Make sure to enjoy them hot.

At Divya's Kitchen we serve Nori-Cheese Sticks as an appetizer along with Ayurvedic "Ketchup" (page 173), but you can pair them with another spicy sauce.

10 ounces pressed paneer cheese
 (page 205; made from ½ gallon milk)

2 toasted nori sheets

BATTER

¼ cup (25 grams) oat flour

¼ cup (33 grams) besan or garbanzo flour

1 small green Indian or Thai chile, seeded
 and finely minced

½ teaspoon salt

¼ teaspoon ground coriander

¼ teaspoon ground turmeric

¼ teaspoon Protein Digestive Masala
 (page 233)

⅛ teaspoon freshly ground black pepper

Tiny pinch of asafoetida

2 tablespoons minced fresh dill

¼ teaspoon fresh lime juice

2 tablespoons melted ghee

To prep the paneer and nori:

1. Cut the paneer into 8 sticks, 2 inches long and ½ inch thick.

2. Cut the nori sheets into 8 equal pieces— each piece just big enough to encompass one cheese stick, about 2 inches long and 3 inches wide.

To prepare the batter:

3. In a small bowl, combine the flours, chile, salt, coriander, turmeric, masala, pepper, and asafoetida, and mix well. Fold in the dill and lime juice, then, stirring with a whisk,

Opposite: Nori-Cheese Sticks, Ayurvedic "Ketchup"

gradually add ½ cup room temperature water and combine to a smooth consistency. (The batter should be thinner than that of pancakes.)

To form and cook the cheese sticks:

4. Fill a small bowl with cold water. Dip a piece of nori in the water for a second, then spread it on a flat surface (the rougher side facing up, the 2-inch side closer to you). Place one cheese stick on top of the nori, positioning its length to align with the 2-inch side of the nori. Then tightly roll the nori over the cheese until you can "seal" the remaining edge of the nori to the cheese stick (similar to rolling sushi). Repeat this process to wrap the remaining cheese sticks.

5. Heat a cast-iron griddle over medium heat. Have the melted ghee ready, and add it to the griddle just before adding the battered cheese sticks.

6. Dip each cheese stick in the batter, making sure to cover all of its sides, then quickly remove it and place it onto the hot griddle. Repeat with the remaining cheese sticks.

7. Panfry, rotating the cheese sticks to help them develop a golden crust on all sides, about 5 minutes. The cast-iron gets hotter as cooking continues, so make sure to moderate the heat. If your ghee starts smoking, turn off the heat for a minute, then turn it back on at a lower setting.

8. Serve hot, with your sauce of choice.

paneer cheese

MAKES about 1½ cups • **PREP:** 3 minutes for soft cheese; 20 minutes for pressed cheese •
COOK: about 15 minutes • **GF** • **YEAR-ROUND**

In *What to Eat for How You Feel*, I give great detail on the process and trouble-shooting of making paneer. Here is an abbreviated version of that recipe. It is always best to bring milk to a boil over a lower heat, as it allows the milk proteins to break down slowly, making them easier to digest.

½ gallon raw or whole
   non-homogenized milk

3 to 4 tablespoons fresh lime juice or
   ½ cup plain buttermilk or yogurt

1. Add just enough water to cover the bottom of a 4-quart heavy-bottomed saucepan (this will protect the milk from scorching). Pour in the milk, and bring to a simmer over low heat.

2. As soon as the milk starts to rise, add the lime juice, and stir gently until the milk forms clumpy curds and separates from the yellowish whey. Turn off the heat.

3. Strain the curds through a mesh strainer (if you need soft cheese) or through a strainer lined with a cheesecloth (if you need pressed cheese); discard the whey. Rinse briefly with cold water to wash away the acidity from the whey. If you're making soft cheese, it is ready at this point.

To make pressed cheese:

4. Gather the corners of the cheesecloth, making sure that the cheese is tightly enclosed within it, then gently twist the cloth to squeeze out the excess liquid.

5. Place the tightly wrapped cheese on a smooth, flat surface, and press the bundled curds with something heavy, like a cast-iron pan or pot. A tofu press works really well for making pressed cheese made from up to 2 gallons of milk. Press for 15 to 20 minutes, until the cheese is firm enough to hold itself together but is still soft and spongy.

6. Unwrap and use as directed in a recipe.

7. Store (either version) in an airtight container in the refrigerator for up to three days.

marinated paneer cheese, two ways

SERVES 4 ● PREP: 5 minutes (with already made paneer cheese) ●
COOK AND MARINATE: at least 30 minutes ● GF ● YEAR-ROUND ● Photograph on page 103

This side dish is usually the first to disappear from the buffet table, be it at home or at a dining event I'm hosting. There is something very attractive about chunks of cheese marinating in a spicy broth—you're just drawn to their glowing yellow color, and when you bite into their soft and succulent nature, you feel a tender squeak between your teeth as if it's whispering the truth of nourishment to your body.

Marinated Paneer Cheese is an excellent protein addition to cooked vegetables, leafy greens, salads, or breads.

INDIAN FLAVOR

2 teaspoons ghee

4 cloves

Two 2-inch cinnamon sticks

½ teaspoon cumin seeds

2 teaspoons salt

1 mace lace (optional)

½ teaspoon ground coriander

½ teaspoon ground turmeric

½ teaspoon freshly ground black pepper

Tiny pinch of asafoetida

MEDITERRANEAN FLAVOR

2 teaspoons ghee

4 black cardamom pods

4 whole dried garcinia indica or garcinia cambogia fruits (optional)

½ teaspoon cumin seeds

2 teaspoons salt

½ teaspoon ground coriander

½ teaspoon ground turmeric

¼ teaspoon freshly ground black pepper

Tiny pinch of asafoetida

10 ounces pressed paneer cheese (page 205, from ½ gallon milk), cut into ¾-inch cubes (1½ cups)

GARNISH

1 tablespoon chopped fresh parsley or a few fresh oregano leaves

For the Indian flavor:

In a 2-quart saucepan or sauté pan, heat the ghee over medium-low heat. Toast the cloves, cinnamon sticks, and cumin seeds for about 10 seconds, then add the salt, mace, coriander, turmeric, pepper, and asafoetida, and toast for a few seconds.

For the Mediterranean flavor:

In a 2-quart saucepan or sauté pan, heat the ghee over medium-low heat. Toast the cardamom pods, garnica fruit, and cumin seeds for about 10 seconds, then add salt, coriander, turmeric, pepper, and asafoetida, and toast for a few seconds.

To finish both flavors:

1. Toast all the spices for another 10 seconds or so, until they release their aroma. Gently stir in the paneer and then 2½ cups hot water (the water should be fully covering the paneer). Bring to a boil, then turn off the heat, cover, and let the paneer marinate and plump for at least 20 minutes or up to 2 hours.

2. Just before serving, reheat the marinated paneer, and use a slotted spoon to serve the cheese pieces without the liquid. Garnish with parsley.

GHEE

I often wonder why the ancient Ayurvedic doctors hailed cultured ghee as the best cooking fat, yet today so many people don't know about it. This superior clarified butter has probably lost its glory throughout the centuries as cheaper cooking oil alternatives have flooded the food market. Nevertheless, cultured ghee continues to be the healthiest source of edible fat for humans. It is my number one food for promoting longevity, and I cook with it every day. If you are accustomed to cooking with butter, you will not be disappointed by cultured ghee because it will deliver the same enticing buttery flavor, but it will feel much lighter in your body.

Ghee is an exceptional carrier, taking herbs and fat-soluble vitamins (A, D, E, and K) to their desired cellular targets in the body. The ancient doctors recognized its bioavailability and used it in thousands of Ayurvedic herbal formulations.

Modern studies confirm that cultured ghee is the food with the highest source of butyric acid, the component that nourishes the gut microbiome, wards off bad bacteria, seals leaky gut, and boosts natural stem cell production. Cultured ghee from grass-fed cows is also very rich in conjugated linoleic acid (CLA), which helps reduce body fat. Yes, cultured ghee can help you lose weight! Even though it is a saturated fat, it does not raise bad cholesterol levels. Moreover, cultured ghee has shown to slow down aging and cellular degeneration.

Cultured ghee is a multistep process: first heavy cream is cultured and fermented into a thick yogurt, then it is churned into butter, and finally it is cooked into ghee (see recipe in *What to Eat for How You Feel*). This cultured form of ghee has superior attributes and healing properties compared to uncultured ghee, which is the predominant type on the market today. Cultured ghee is lighter to digest and does not build unnecessary fat tissue. Below I present the properties of cultured ghee.

SANSKRIT NAME ● *Ghrita*

AYURVEDIC ATTRIBUTES

TASTE ● sweet

QUALITIES: ● heavy, oily

METABOLIC EFFECT ● cooling

POST-DIGESTIVE EFFECT ● sweet

DOSHA EFFECTS ● balances all three doshas, although Kapha needs less of it

HEALING BENEFITS ● restores vitality, enhances vision, kindles *agni*, lubricates the channels in the body, prolongs life, nourishes the brain, supports healthy hormone production, and more

SOURCING

● Not only does your health benefit most from making your own ghee but it is also more economical. In the US, you can find several brands of cultured ghee, including my own brand, Divya's. We make organic, cultured ghee following the traditional Ayurvedic recipe, and I stand by its high quality. However, I encourage you to try multiple brands and see which one you like the most. Making cultured ghee is a lengthy process; that's why it is more expensive than conventional ghee, which is derived from sweet butter (skipping the cream-culturing process).

CONTINUED

- The best quality ghee is made from organic cream that comes from happy grass-fed A2 cows. As a saturated fat, ghee solidifies at temperatures below 90°F. The healthy color of hardened ghee is a light to rich yellow, and when melted, the ghee should look like liquid gold. Discard ghee of whitish color, which is a sign that it has gone rancid.

- Ghee is a precious substance with a long shelf life. Protect it by keeping it in a dark and dry place (do not refrigerate it), and always use a dry spoon to scoop it out of the jar. Even a drop of liquid can spoil the ghee.

SEASON

- Ghee can be used throughout the year. Increase consumption in the fall and winter to counteract the dryness in the environment—it will moisturize your body on the inside. Use less of it in the spring and summer.

DIGESTIBILITY

- Cultured ghee kindles *agni*, so it is a digestive by itself, but it still remains a fat that the body needs to break down. Solid ghee is clogging and bile-thickening; therefore, food with ghee should be eaten warm.

COOKING TIPS

- Ghee has a high smoke point of 485°F and is suitable for all methods of cooking, including panfrying and roasting.

- Always heat ghee over low to medium heat, and be watchful in order to protect it from smoking or burning (if that happens, discard it and start again).

- Do not reuse ghee that is left over after cooking it in any way.

- You can use ghee instead of butter in all recipes. The slight exception is with pie dough—ghee will work, but the pie crust will be less flaky.

COOK WITH GHEE WHEN YOU WANT TO

- feel grounded and satiated,
- calm your nervous system,
- increase physical and mental stamina,
- enhance the complexion and glow of your skin,
- slow down aging, and/or
- improve your memory and learning ability.

CAUTION • Do not use ghee if you have chronic liver or kidney disease, if you are experiencing an alcohol hangover, or if you have a sciatica pain attack.

quick cultured ghee

MAKES 2 cups (16 ounces) ● PREP: 3 minutes ● COOK: about 30 minutes ● GF ● YEAR-ROUND

In *What to Eat for How You Feel*, I explain in great detail how to make cultured ghee from scratch. In this recipe, I take you through the last step: cooking ghee using store-bought cultured butter.

Making ghee is a good practice of mindfulness—you have to be around it, observe it, and protect it from burning. To increase vibrational potency, make your ghee on a day of the full moon, and play a recording of sacred music while cooking it.

1 pound (2 cups) organic unsalted cultured butter

1. Place the butter in a 3-quart heavy-bottomed pot, and turn on the burner to the lowest possible setting. Stir occasionally as the butter melts and starts to bubble. (To speed up melting time, cut the butter into pieces before adding it to the pot.) As the butter simmers, its contents will separate: the milk solids will sink to the bottom, and the water will rise to the top as foam. Stir occasionally to help the water evaporate. The key is to simmer the butter over low heat, which will protect it from burning before it fully clarifies.

2. When the solids have more or less settled to the bottom (as opposed to floating around), stop stirring from the bottom up. Let the milk fat solids rest at the bottom. At this point in time, you'll also notice that the butterfat begins to lose its cloudiness. This is because the temperature of the butter rises faster due to a decrease in water content, therefore clarifying the butter.

3. The ghee is ready when the butter oil is a clear, amber color, and the solids on the bottom of the pan are a consistent golden-brown color. You should be able to clearly see the bottom of the pan. If the solids are mostly tan, continue to simmer for a few more minutes. If the solids have become black, you've scorched the ghee and, regretfully, you will have to discard it.

4. Fold a cheesecloth into 8 layers (2 layers if using a flour sack towel), and place it in a strainer atop a mixing bowl.

5. At this point, make sure all utensils that the ghee comes in contact with are completely dry, as moisture will spoil the ghee. Carefully but quickly pour or ladle the hot ghee through the cheesecloth; do not squeeze the cheesecloth to hurry the process or try to get more ghee out of the solids. Discard the strained solids. To clean and reuse the cheesecloth, soak it in boiling hot water with soap; handwash while the soapy water is still warm.

6. Let the ghee cool for a few minutes, allowing any air molecules to dissipate. Pour the ghee into a glass jar. Put on the lid only when the jar has cooled to room temperature. Store in a dark and dry place, such as a cabinet or a drawer. Your ghee will be good for six months.

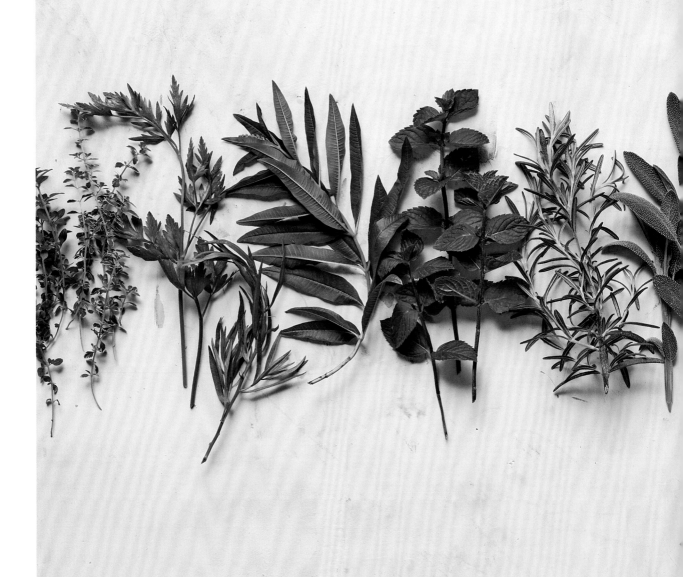

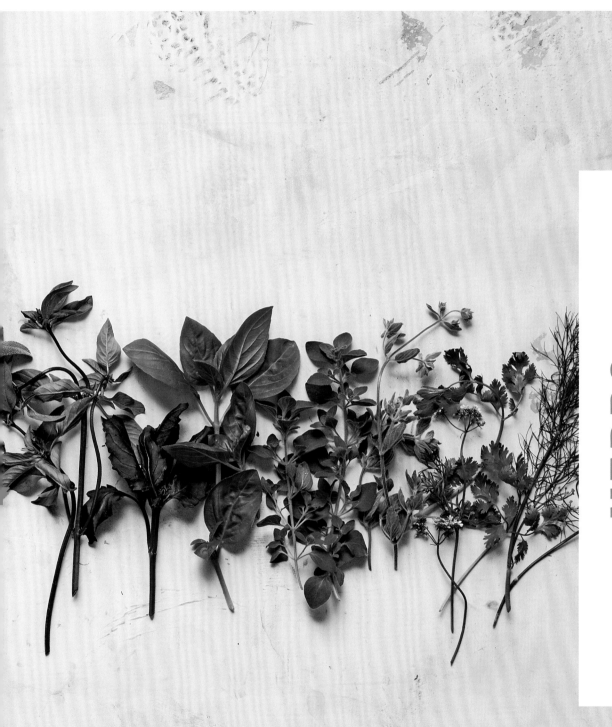

HERBS

HERBS

I can't properly express the joy I feel when I grow my own culinary herbs. Whenever my husband, Prentiss, and I choose a residence, we make sure that there is at least one balcony or rooftop where I can line up my planters and grow the herbaceous plants I love to cook with. From spring through late fall, basil, parsley, thyme, dill, oregano, rosemary, curry leaves, tarragon, sage, lemon verbena, mint, and moringa beautify our house and serve as my cooking companions.

Often used to garnish our meals, these herbs excite our senses with an appealing green color and the freshest flavors. Additionally, growing my own herbs allows me the flexibility to use the exact quantity I need when I need it—for example, just 1 tablespoon of dill to test a recipe—without worrying that a whole bunch will go bad before I have the chance to use it all. In turn, this saves me money and refrigeration space! Before my garden herbs go to seed, I dehydrate any excess and use them in my meals throughout the winter, until the next growing season is underway. My herb balcony garden is my humble attempt to live more attuned to nature. I dream of one day having a spacious teaching garden in

a rural environment where I can cultivate herbs, fruits, and vegetables. It will be a place for the public to visit and connect with ingredients from their origins in the soil to their beautiful offering on the table. Until then, I'll keep up my herb balcony garden in New York City.

Culinary herbs predominantly consist of the leaves of medicinal plants. For therapeutic remedies, Ayurveda would often accept all parts of a plant—roots, stems, bark, leaves, fruits, seeds, or flowers. In this section, I will focus on herbs for cooking. Irish moss is a seaweed, but I've included it in this section because its rich mineral content and binding properties act like a healing herb in my recipes.

SOURCING

- Fresh herbs are available at farmers markets and grocery stores. Select leaves that are crisp and of a darker green color. Dried herbs can be purchased in grocery stores and online specialty stores. Always check their expiration date. Herbs spoil quickly, and conventional farmers spray the fresh ones with a lot of pesticides (especially mint) and irradiate the dry ones. Organic herbs are your healthiest choice.

- To store fresh herbs, wrap them in a wet kitchen towel or paper towel, and store them in a biodegradable bag in the refrigerator drawer; use them within a few days.

- To store dried herbs, keep them in airtight containers placed away from light and humidity.

SEASON

- Whether grown indoors, outdoors, or in greenhouses, fresh herbs are available all year round.

COOKING TIPS

- Substitute 1 teaspoon dry herbs for 1 tablespoon fresh herbs.

- To minimize oxidation, use a sharp knife to slice the fresh leaves into thin ribbons rather than mincing them.

- Add dried herbs at the beginning of cooking and fresh herbs as a garnish or in the final stage of cooking.

Learn more about specific herbs in the following entries.

ALOE VERA

In my younger years, I had only associated aloe vera with skin care products, until I realized that I can actually cook with it. Of course, it is great for your skin, too. Maybe you've been advised to cover a burn with the juicy part of an aloe leaf or rest the leaves on your eyes to reduce swelling and dark circles. Ayurveda has used aloe for centuries and outlines so many healing properties that I have to list them separately from its other attributes.

BOTANICAL NAME ● *Aloe Vera*

SANSKRIT NAME ● *Kumari*

AYURVEDIC ATTRIBUTES

TASTE ● sweet, bitter

QUALITIES ● moist, slimy

METABOLIC EFFECT ● cooling

POST-DIGESTIVE EFFECT ● pungent

DOSHA EFFECTS ● useful in diseases caused by Vata, Pitta, and Kapha imbalances

SOURCING

● For internal consumption, use the large, mature leaves of aloe, not the small leaves growing as a potted ornamental plant. Fresh aloe leaves are sold in a lot of grocery stores. You might also be able to find them in farmers markets in California and other subtropical regions.

SEASON

● Aloe vera grows all year round in hot climates, but the leaves need to grow for at least eight months before they are harvested.

HEALING BENEFITS FOR EXTERNAL USE

● Aloe's anti-inflammatory properties work wonders when applied as a poultice on inflamed skin.

● Apply drops of fresh aloe juice in eyes affected by conjunctivitis.

● Spread aloe pulp on gauze, and apply it locally for headaches and eye problems.

● Aloe vera is a universal remedy for soothing topical burns. Mostly water soluble, aloe offers refreshing coolness to the first layer of the skin, which holds moisture, thus enhancing the skin's luster and complexion.

HEALING BENEFITS FOR INTERNAL USE

● Aloe vera juice supports the digestive system by increasing the digestive fire, thus helping with a loss of appetite or abdominal colic, when taken in small doses. It increases the secretions in the small intestine and promotes peristalsis in the large intestine. It also has antidotal properties (used to neutralize or counteract the effects of poison). Since aloe's action is slow, its purgative and laxative properties take effect ten to twelve hours after intake.

● In the cardiovascular system, aloe helps purify the blood, support the plasma, and cool the liver. In combination with turmeric, it is used to reduce inflammation on an enlarged spleen.

● Aloe supports the reproductive fluids in the urogenital system. By virtue of being moist and slippery, aloe promotes the secretion of semen and acts as an aphrodisiac. It is also a known diuretic.

● Aloe vera also supports muscles, bones, and fat. It is useful in treating chronic fevers.

● A single dose for internal use is 2 to 4 tablespoons of aloe vera leaf juice, or as recommended by an Ayurvedic doctor.

CAUTION

● A large dose of aloe is a purgative and helps expel parasites, but when taken in excess, it may cause digestive discomfort, anal congestion, and sometimes internal bleeding. Use large doses of aloe vera juice only under the direction of an Ayurvedic doctor.

● Intake of aloe vera may interact with medications; therefore, please consult with your medical doctor before consuming the herb.

to extract the pulp from an aloe leaf:

1. Wash the aloe leaf.

2. Cut off the bottom two inches of the base and the top two inches of the tip; retain for other uses (e.g., skin care, eyes).

3. Lay the leaf on the cutting board and, using a sharp knife, carefully cut off the two thorny long edges of the leaf.

4. Depending on its length, cut the leaf across into two or three shorter pieces.

5. Stand each piece vertically and cut it in half to expose the most amount (largest surface area) of inner pulp.

6. On each half, use the knife to make multiple grid-like cuts into the pulp. Use a spoon to scrape out the chunks of pulp, but don't scrape too deep into the leaf, as that part is bitter. It's slimy, yes, very slimy and slippery. Don't be put off by it—remember that it's good for you and keep going (the sliminess will disappear after blending).

aloe vera mint cooler

MAKES about 6 cups ● **PREP:** about 15 minutes ● **GF, DF** ● **SUMMER** ● Photograph on page 129

This is the perfect cooling and hydrating drink for a hot summer day. The aloe is hard to detect in taste, but it lends a delicate silkiness in your mouth as you sip on it.

This beverage feels so good, you can almost hear your body saying, "Yes, yes, thank you!" Think of this drink as a restorative tonic that can help you bounce back from physical weakness. If you are an athlete, Aloe Vera Mint Cooler is your homemade superior electrolyte drink. We serve it at Divya's Kitchen during the summer.

½ cup fresh aloe vera pulp, from 1 aloe leaf (see sidebar)

¼ cup raw cane sugar

¼ cup fresh lime juice

¼ cup chopped fresh mint leaves

¼ teaspoon salt (Soma Salt is best in this recipe)

⅛ teaspoon toasted ground cumin

1. In a blender, blend the aloe vera pulp and sugar to a smooth consistency.

2. Add 5 cups filtered or spring water, the lime juice, mint, salt, and cumin, and blend well.

3. Chill and serve. Store covered in the refrigerator for up to 24 hours.

BASIL

I have yet to meet a person who does not like basil. Is it the sweet aroma or the association with our favorite Italian food that draws us to this ancient herb? Basil is an intrinsic part of many world cuisines, not only Italian. I use it to garnish my Indian-style kitchari, Puerto Rican–flavored stew, or Bulgarian-style roasted vegetables.

Culinary basil is of several varieties, each distinct in aroma and color. On the same plant, the intensity of leaf flavor changes with growing conditions and the stage of harvesting. I've noticed that the leaves of a young basil plant are sweeter, and the longer they remain attached to the growing stem, the more pungent they become. Hydroponically grown basil is quite mild in flavor.

Do not confuse culinary basil with holy basil, a.k.a. *tulasi*. The two herbs are cousins, but have different medicinal properties.

BOTANICAL NAME • *Ocimum basilicum*
SANSKRIT NAME • *Barbari*

AYURVEDIC ATTRIBUTES

TASTE • sweet, pungent, or astringent (depending on the variety and maturity)
QUALITIES • light, penetrating, causes dryness
METABOLIC EFFECT • cooling or mildly heating
POST-DIGESTIVE EFFECT • pungent
DOSHA EFFECTS • slightly increases Pitta, mitigates Vata and Kapha
HEALING BENEFITS • enhances digestion, improves the taste of food, supports the heart

FOR SOURCING, SEASON, AND COOKING TIPS, SEE RECOMMENDATIONS UNDER HERBS (PAGE 213).

DIGESTIBILITY

- Basil is a digestive aid—you do not need help to digest it.

EAT BASIL WHEN YOU NEED TO

- resolve cold symptoms,
- relieve menstrual cramps,
- digest heavy or clogging foods,
- reduce bloating and gas,
- reverse constipation, and/or
- heal a whooping cough.

basil-parsley pesto

MAKES ⅔ cup ● **PREP:** 15 minutes ● **GF, DF** ● **FALL** ● Photograph on pages 53 and 71

In Italian, *pesto* means "pounded." Traditionally the ingredients are crushed in a large mortar with a pestle, which most of us don't have in our kitchens today. I use a food processor, but with caution—I "pulse" frequently to achieve a coarse texture. I prefer this chunkier appearance and mouthfeel over a smoother consistency because it gives more of a bite, and it looks beautiful as a garnish.

This vibrant green pesto tastes fresh and perky, and it serves as a digestive to the heavier dishes it usually accompanies. Therefore, I much prefer (any) pesto to be without Parmesan cheese, because this kind of aged cheese leaves me with a dull feeling in my stomach, negating the digestive properties of the sauce.

Basil-Parsley Pesto goes well with Minestrone (page 51), Sesame Crackers (page 68), Asparagus Pizza (page 125), and more. Of course, you can use it with pasta or bread. At Divya's Kitchen we serve it with our Lasagna, Carrot Risotto, and Vegetable Bread (page 70).

½ cup olive oil, divided

⅛ teaspoon asafoetida

¼ cup walnuts or pine nuts

2 cups packed chopped fresh basil leaves (about 3 ounces)

½ cup packed chopped fresh parsley leaves (no stems) (about ¾ ounce)

2 teaspoons fresh lime juice

¾ teaspoon salt

1. In a small skillet, heat ¼ cup of the olive oil over low heat, add the asafoetida, and cook for 5 to 10 seconds. Turn off the heat.

2. Place the nuts in a food processor, and pulse a few times to create a fine chop. Add the basil, parsley, lime juice, salt, and both the seasoned and plain olive oil. Continue to pulse to a consistency of your liking.

3. Serve immediately or store refrigerated in an airtight container for up to one week. Take it out of the fridge 30 minutes before serving to let it warm up to room temperature.

CILANTRO

Cilantro is one herb that I did not grow up with. Although it can thrive in Bulgaria, it is not cultivated much there because it is foreign to the local cuisine. Living in India, I fell in love with cilantro and learned how to use it.

The cilantro plant and its seed, coriander, are one of the oldest and most popular herbs and spices in the world. Ayurveda applies them extensively in cleansing and Pitta-reducing protocols.

BOTANICAL NAME ● *Coriandrum sativum*
SANSKRIT NAME ● *Dhanyakam*

Cilantro (Coriander Leaf)

AYURVEDIC ATTRIBUTES

TASTE ● astringent, bitter, pungent
QUALITIES ● light to digest
METABOLIC EFFECT ● cooling
POST-DIGESTIVE EFFECT ● sweet
DOSHA EFFECTS ● balancing for all three doshas
HEALING BENEFITS ● chelates heavy metals, binds chemical toxins, stops bleeding

Coriander Seed

AYURVEDIC ATTRIBUTES

TASTE ● sweet
QUALITIES ● light to digest
METABOLIC EFFECT ● cooling
POST-DIGESTIVE EFFECT ● sweet
DOSHA EFFECTS ● balances all three doshas

HEALING BENEFITS ● reduces fever, acts as a diuretic, binds hot and acidic toxins, supports absorption of nutrients in the colon, tonifies the bone marrow and nerves, stimulates digestion without aggravating Pitta

FOR SOURCING, SEASON, AND COOKING TIPS, SEE RECOMMENDATIONS UNDER HERBS (PAGE 213) AND SPICES (PAGE 231).

EAT CORIANDER/CILANTRO WHEN YOU NEED TO

- detox,
- cool down from feeling overheated,
- eliminate kidney stones,
- reduce gas and bloating,
- soothe an irritated gut,
- clear a urinary tract infection, and/or
- stop colic pain in your baby if you're breastfeeding (see sidebar).

coriander-fennel tea for nursing mothers

If you're breastfeeding, drink this tea to relieve colic pains in your baby.

Bring 2 cups filtered or spring water to a boil. Add ½ teaspoon coriander seeds and ½ teaspoon fennel seeds. Turn off the heat, steep for 10 minutes, then strain. Sip it slowly, finishing the tea within two hours (you may store it in a thermos during this time to keep it hot).

green tahini sauce

MAKES 1 cup ● PREP: 10 minutes ● GF, DF ● YEAR-ROUND ● Photograph on pages 85 and 155

This vibrant green sauce makes you expand on the inside—you will really feel it.

Serve Green Tahini Sauce with Simple Kitchari (page 94), Celery Root and Taro Pancakes (page 153), Kulthi Lentil Stew, Puerto Rican Style (page 81), Braised Purple Cabbage (page 117), and more.

⅓ cup roasted tahini

1 ounce cilantro with stems, coarsely chopped (about 2 loosely packed cups)

1 medium green Indian or Thai chile, seeded and chopped

1 tablespoon chopped fresh ginger

2 tablespoons fresh lime juice, or to taste

½ teaspoon Warming Masala (page 233)

¼ teaspoon salt, or to taste

⅛ teaspoon ground cinnamon

1. Place all the ingredients and ½ cup water in a small blender, and blend to a creamy consistency. Adjust the salt and lime juice to your liking.

2. Store in a covered jar in the refrigerator for up to three days.

GREEN INDIAN OR THAI CHILES

I am one of those people who start coughing and sneezing by smelling a mere hint of any kind of chile. It must be some genetic imperfection. When I told Vaidya Mishra (a chile lover) about my reaction, he laughed and said, "The more you advance in Ayurveda, the more you will be able to tolerate chiles." Thank God he was joking, because by that criterion, my hopes of progress would be crushed for life.

Chiles are a relatively recently cultivated herb. They were discovered in South America some five hundred years ago, and since then, they have quickly infiltrated every cuisine in the world. Today we know of several hundred chile varieties, in fresh and dried forms.

Among the members of the capsicum family, red chiles are cautioned against in the Shaka Vansiya Ayurveda lineage. Instead, it favors small green chiles. Different types grow in different parts of the world. Vaidya R. K. Mishra recommended green Indian chiles or Thai (a.k.a. bird's eye) chiles. These ones are small, thin, less fleshy, and very pungent—much more piquant than a jalapeño but less hot than a habanero. Chiles in general create dryness in the body, but green chiles have a bit more moisture and thus are a bit less drying to the lining of the stomach compared to red, orange, or yellow colored chiles. The unripe fruits of the Thai chile plant are green, and if not harvested at that stage, they continue to mature, changing to a red color, with an increased level of heat.

BOTANICAL NAME ● *Capsicum annuum*

SANSKRIT NAME ● *Katuvira*

AYURVEDIC ATTRIBUTES

TASTE ● pungent

QUALITIES ● light, sharp, penetrating, causes dryness

METABOLIC EFFECT ● heating

POST-DIGESTIVE EFFECT ● pungent

DOSHA EFFECTS ● aggravates Pitta, balances Kapha and (when in small amounts) Vata

HEALING BENEFITS ● acts as a cardiac stimulant, increases libido, creates excess salivation, acts as a diuretic (if taken in small amounts), opens the body's channels

SOURCING

● Look for green Indian or Thai chiles in your local grocer or at specialty Indian or other Asian grocery stores. Select chiles that are dark green, firm, and shiny. Store them refrigerated in a small, covered container.

● If you cannot find green Indian or Thai chiles, select a green variety that comes close to the description above.

SEASON

● Because chiles are very heating, use them more in the colder seasons (including parts of the fall and spring) and less in the summer.

DIGESTIBILITY

Chiles increase *agni* and act as a digestive aid. However, to enjoy them in a balancing way, follow these recommendations:

- Don't eat them raw (see cooking ideas below).
- Add a cooling spice, such as coriander, green cardamom, or fennel, to offset their heating potency.
- Chiles are in the nightshade family—keep that in mind if you have nightshade sensitivities.

COOKING TIPS

- When seeding and mincing chiles, protect your skin from burning by wearing gloves or coating your hands with oil. After touching chiles, wash your hands with water and soap, and do not rub your eyes.
- If you feel a burning sensation on an area of your skin that touched chiles, wash it off with soap, and apply coconut oil, fresh aloe vera, cucumber, or milk.
- To reduce the sharp pungency of a chile, scrape away the seeds and soft membrane. You might notice that I recommend seeded and minced chiles in all my recipes— prepared this way, I find them to lend a more "elegant" pungency, one that is felt on the tongue without creating a burning sensation in the throat.
- Ways to cook chiles: toast them in oil, and add them to a boiling soup; roast, pickle, or marinate them.

EAT GREEN CHILES WHEN YOU NEED TO

- increase *agni,*
- digest heavy or clogging foods,
- move out stagnant *ama,*
- improve circulation,
- induce sweating,
- enhance fat burning/lose weight,
- purge parasites, and/or
- dissolve cold symptoms or phlegm.

DO NOT EAT GREEN (OR ANY) CHILES WHEN YOU ARE EXPERIENCING

- a burning sensation anywhere in your body,
- a hot liver condition,
- gut irritation or inflammation,
- excessive dryness,
- eye redness or dry eyes,
- hot flashes, and/or
- other types of Pitta imbalance.

CAUTION ● Overuse of chile can cause muscle weakness, dizziness, hemorrhage, or kidney damage.

marinated green chiles

MAKES about 1½ cups • **PREP:** 10 minutes • **COOK:** 10 minutes • **GF, DF** • **FALL-WINTER-SPRING**

Here is a way high Pitta individuals can enjoy chile peppers! Vaidya Mishra personally taught this recipe to my dear friend Kandarpa Bhuckory, who transformed it to the recipe you see below. He explained that the preparation of the chiles in ghee and oil, as shown below, reduces the overheating effect that many people experience. Leave the chiles whole, with their stems removed—they will last longer this way, acting like a pickle. I find it interesting that the heat of the chiles transfers to the oil the longer the chiles marinate. The oil absorbs the flavor of the chiles, and it then serves as a pungent condiment. If you're cooking a meal for people who can tolerate different levels of heat, omit any chile in the dish, and just serve Marinated Green Chiles on the side. A few drops of its olive oil will make a dish pungent without changing the dish's flavor, color, or texture.

This recipe is a condiment—add a little bit to your meal, taste, and then decide if you need more.

1 cup olive oil, divided

20 fresh curry leaves, washed and patted dry

1 teaspoon cumin seeds

1 tablespoon salt

1 teaspoon ground turmeric

1 cup green Indian or Thai chiles, stems removed, washed, and patted dry

2 tablespoons Protein Digestive Masala (page 233)

3 tablespoons fresh lime juice

1. In a medium skillet, heat ¼ cup olive oil over low heat. Add the curry leaves and cook until lightly crisp. Add the cumin seeds and toast until they darken a shade, then add the salt and turmeric. Add the chiles, increase the heat to medium, and cook for 5 minutes, stirring occasionally. Add the masala and continue to cook for 2 minutes. The chiles will make popping sounds, and some of them may burst. Their green color should change from bright to dull. Turn off the heat.

2. Allow the chiles to cool for 5 minutes, then stir in the remaining ¾ cup olive oil and lime juice.

3. Store the marinated chiles in an airtight glass jar. You can eat them right away or, for a stronger flavor, marinate them in the closed jar at room temperature for two to three days and then refrigerate them for up to three months. Leave them out at room temperature for 30 minutes before serving. You may also choose to not eat the chiles and just use the infused oil as a garnish or in a dressing or chutney.

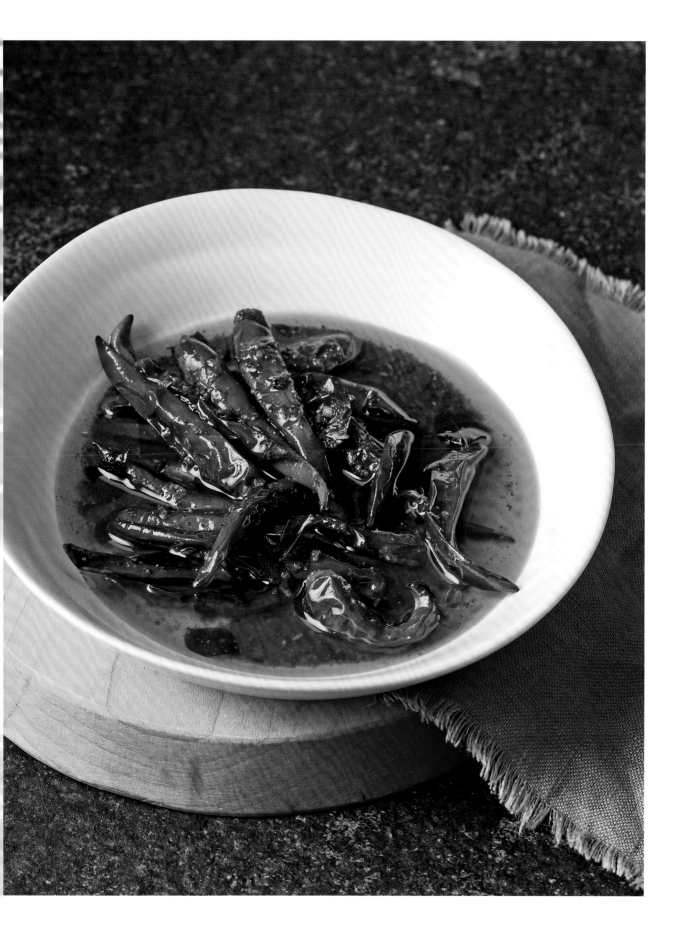

IRISH MOSS

I discovered Irish moss a decade ago, when dining at Café Gratitude in the San Francisco Bay Area. I was astonished at how seaweed could be a key ingredient in creating gelatinous vegan desserts that held their shape and tasted so delicious. I immediately purchased Café Gratitude's cookbooks and started experimenting with the moss.

Even though seaweed is not mentioned in the Ayurvedic classical texts, I've decided to profile it because I want to show you how to create attractive mousse or gel-like delights with this most nutritious ingredient. As are all ocean plants, Irish moss is a remarkable source of iodine, vitamin A, and trace minerals.

BOTANICAL NAME ● *Chondrus crispus*
SANSKRIT NAME ● Unknown

AYURVEDIC ATTRIBUTES

TASTE ● salty

QUALITIES ● slippery, mobile

METABOLIC EFFECT ● cooling (of soaked moss)

POST-DIGESTIVE EFFECT ● pungent

DOSHA EFFECTS ● balances Vata, okay for Pitta, increases Kapha (of soaked moss)

HEALING BENEFITS ● acts as an antidiuretic, increases thyroid function, acts as a prebiotic food, binds toxins in the blood

SOURCING

● See Sources (page 248) for where to purchase Irish moss in the US.

● For the recipes in this book, you will need the raw, dried, whole Irish moss, not the flakes or powder. It should look like soft, yellowish seaweed clusters covered with sand.

SEASON

● Use Irish moss in the summer or fall and less in the spring and winter.

DIGESTIBILITY

● Soaked and blended moss is easy to digest. Follow the recipe instructions to make sure you prepare Irish moss in a digestible way.

COOKING TIPS

Irish moss comes with a strong sea odor. To eliminate it and make it easy to eat, you must clean and soak it in the following manner:

1. Place the moss in a bowl, and remove any foreign material, such as colored threads, shells, or discolored leaves.

2. Fill the bowl with cold water, and move the moss around to separate the sand. Repeat with fresh water until you can't see any gritty particles at the bottom of the bowl.

3. Place the cleaned leaves in a container with a lid, add cold water (3 inches above the moss), and let the moss soak in the refrigerator for at least 8 hours or up to 4 days.

4. Take it out of the refrigerator 30 minutes before you are ready to use it, discard the soaking water, and rinse the moss thoroughly. It is now ready to use in my recipes.

5. Soak and refrigerate any remaining moss. Discard after 4 days.

EAT IRISH MOSS WHEN YOU NEED TO

● alleviate ulcers,

● restore the lining of your gut,

● strengthen your kidneys,

● regulate your bowels,

● take in mineral-rich foods, and/or

● add more iodine and vitamin A to your diet.

CAUTION ● Do not consume Irish moss if you are allergic to fish or shellfish.

rose chocolate mousse

SERVES 6 ● **SOAK:** 8 hours ● **PREP:** 20 minutes ● **CHILL:** 2 hours ● **GF, DF** ● **SUMMER-FALL** ●
Photograph on page 226

This is based on a vegan raw dessert that I first tasted at Café Gratitude. Years later, I included my "Ayurvedized" version of it on the Divya's Kitchen menu. Cacao and chocolate tend to be clogging foods because they are very dry, acidic, and require strong *agni*. In this recipe, the pink pepper helps digest the cacao, the Irish moss mitigates its dryness and acidity, and the rose water and petals add a subtle aroma and mood-lifting effect. Sweetened only with dates, to me, this dessert is one of the healthiest ways to enjoy chocolate.

2 ounces soaked and well drained Irish moss (see instructions on page 224; from ½ ounce of dried Irish moss), finely chopped

2¼ cups almond or sunflower milk (see page 184), divided

7 ounces pitted dates, finely chopped (about 1 cup)

1½ ounces (⅓ cup + 1 tablespoon) raw cacao powder

3 tablespoons vanilla extract

2 tablespoons rose water

¼ teaspoon salt

⅓ cup melted raw coconut oil

1 tablespoon liquid sunflower lecithin (optional, for consistency)

GARNISHES

2 tablespoons slivered almonds

Pink peppercorns, crushed

Dried rose petals

1. In a high-speed blender, combine the Irish moss, ¾ cup of the almond milk, and ¼ cup water, and blend until very smooth and creamy.

2. Add the remaining 1½ cups almond milk, the dates, cacao, vanilla, rose water, and salt, and blend until very smooth.

3. Add the coconut oil and sunflower lecithin, and continue blending for another 10 seconds, or until all ingredients are well combined. For the correct consistency, it is important to blend the ingredients in the sequence I've described above and not all at once.

4. Line up six dessert cups, each big enough to hold 4 to 6 ounces of liquid. Evenly pour the mousse into the cups. Wipe the cups clean from any dripped chocolate, cover each cup with plastic wrap or a saucer (this will protect the mousse from crusting and absorbing other odors from the refrigerator), and refrigerate for 2 hours, or until the mousse has thickened.

5. This dessert must be served chilled to retain its mousse consistency. Before serving, sprinkle the garnishes on each cup in this order: 1 teaspoon slivered almonds, a pinch of pink pepper, two pinches of rose petals. Store refrigerated for up to three days.

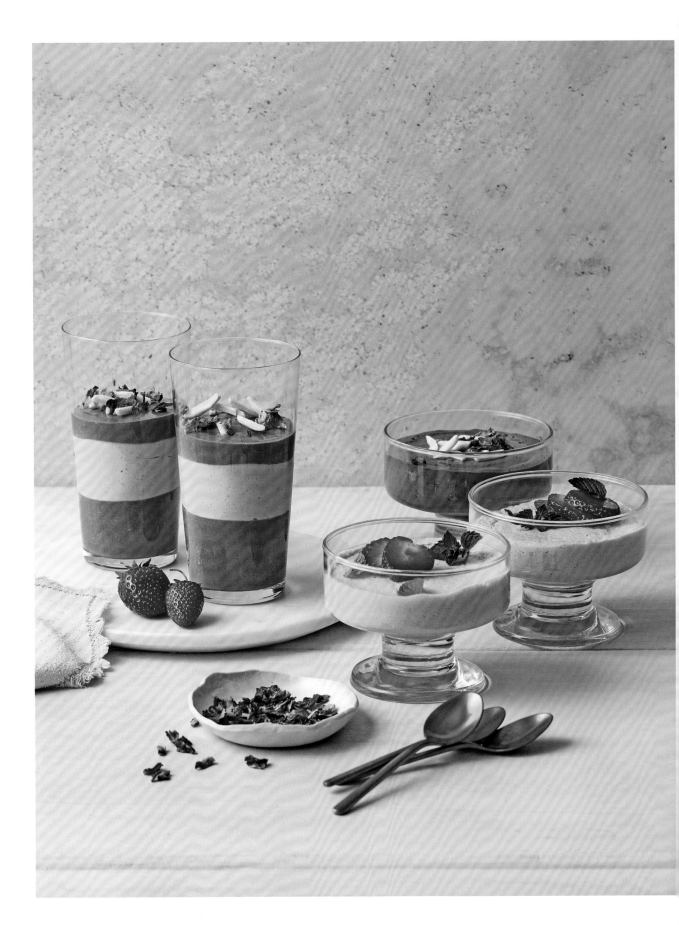

strawberry parfait

SERVES 6 ● SOAK: 8 hours ● PREP: 20 minutes ● CHILL: at least 2 hours or overnight ● GF, DF ●
SPRING-SUMMER

When strawberry season arrives, I often wonder what more I can make with this delectable but fast-spoiling fruit. *Sweet Gratitude*, by Matthew Rogers and Tiziana Alipo Tamborra, gave me a lot of ideas, including this variation of their recipe. It's impressive how light and fluffy this raw dessert is. With its dreamy pink color and green mint garnish, it completely satisfies my senses' desires as well as my childhood love for strawberry ice cream.

For superb consistency, it is best to serve Strawberry Parfait chilled and on the day of making, but you can keep it covered and refrigerated for up to two days.

1 cup almond or sunflower milk
  (see page 184)

2 ounces soaked and drained Irish moss
  (see instructions on page 224; from
  ½ ounce of dried Irish moss), finely minced

3 cups (12 ounces) trimmed and chopped
  strawberries

½ cup maple syrup

2 tablespoons vanilla extract

2 tablespoons fresh lime juice

½ teaspoon ground cardamom

⅛ teaspoon salt

½ cup melted raw coconut oil

2 tablespoons sunflower lecithin
  (optional, for consistency)

GARNISHES

Thinly sliced strawberries

Fresh mint leaves

Opposite: Strawberry Parfait, Rose Chocolate Mousse

1. In a blender, blend the almond milk and Irish moss until very smooth and creamy.

2. Add the strawberries, maple syrup, vanilla, lime juice, cardamom, and salt, and blend to a smooth consistency.

3. Add the coconut oil and sunflower lecithin, and blend briefly, until the ingredients are fully incorporated.

4. Pour into parfait glasses or other small serving bowls. Set in the fridge for at least 2 hours, until the parfait solidifies. Garnish with fresh strawberries and mint leaves.

VARIATION: To make chocolate-strawberry cups, layer the parfait glasses with Chocolate Mousse (page 225) and Strawberry Parfait.

NOTE: Irish moss—also known as sea moss, carrageenan moss, or rock moss—is an Atlantic seaweed varying in color, from whitish to reddish purple; it is in the red algae family. The name *Irish* was probably added during Ireland's famine of the nineteenth century, when the moss became a lifesaving dietary staple for the local population. Today this sea moss can be sourced from many coasts, including Canada, the US, Ireland, Iceland, the Caribbean, and more.

The extract from Irish moss, known as carrageenan, is a common food-industry ingredient used for thickening, gelling, or stabilizing ice cream, beer, yogurt, plant milk, and more. After years of studies and debates on whether carrageenan is safe for human consumption, the FDA stood by its decision to allow it in minimal amounts in food products. Note that the industrially produced carrageenan is an *extract* of sea moss, and as such has different effects than the whole food, which is naturally balanced.

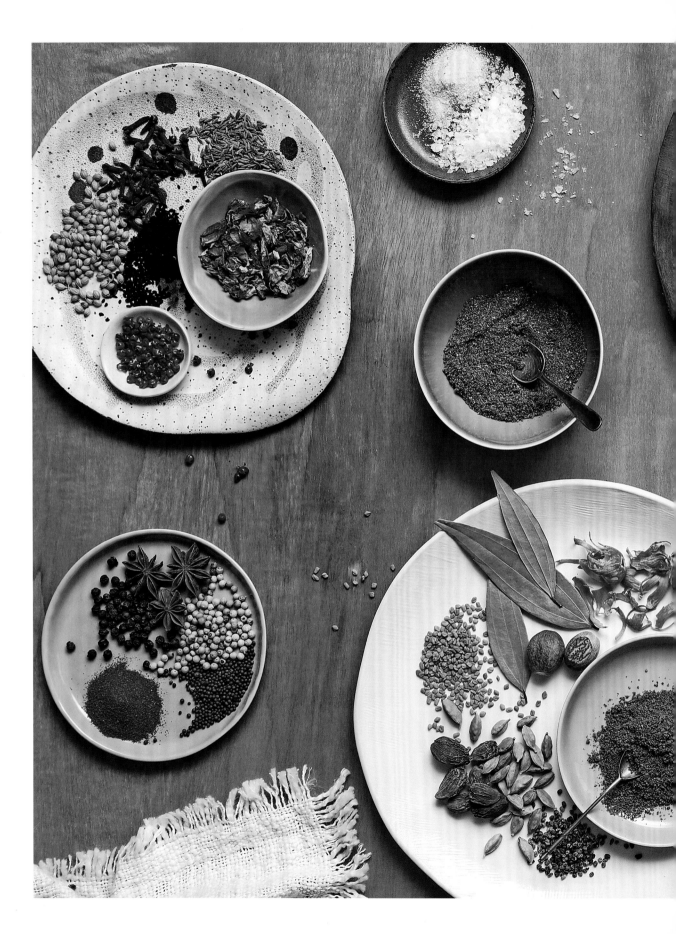

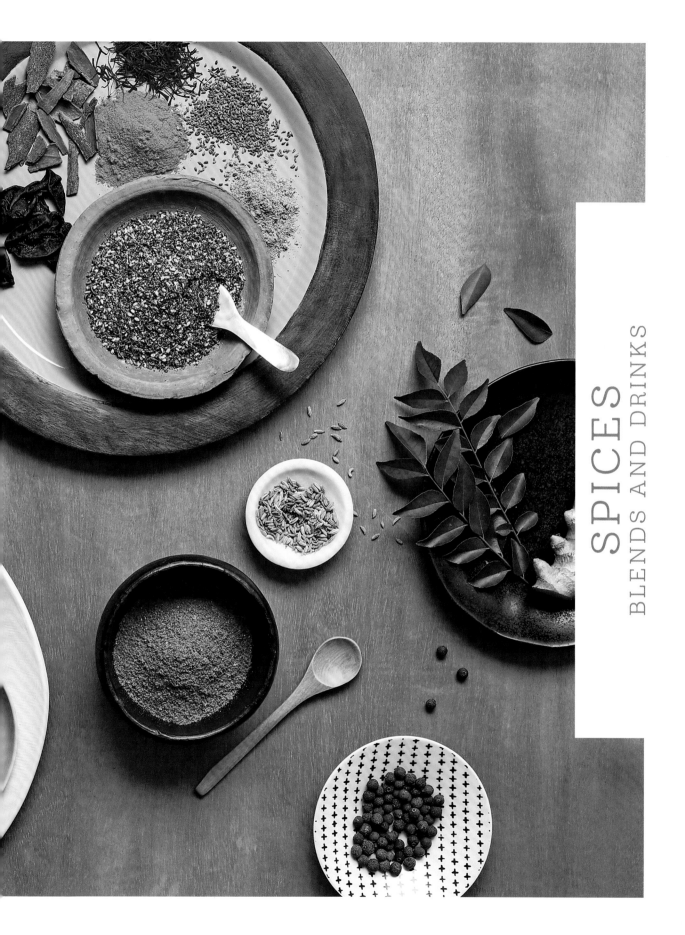

SPICES
BLENDS AND DRINKS

SPICES

When people ask me what is unique about Ayurvedic cooking, I say, "It is the way we use spices." Most spices originate from India and were mentioned in the classical texts, but cooking with them does not mean that the food must taste like Indian cuisine. You will notice this phenomenon throughout the book, as I present recipes adapted from international culinary fare and use spices in all of them.

For example, I season the Stuffed Cabbage Rolls (page 113) with ginger and asafoetida, but they taste very European. The Kulthi Lentil Stew, Puerto Rican Style (page 81) calls for cumin, black cardamom, asafoetida, pepper, coriander, chile, saffron, and more—and it tastes very much like a stew from that island. The Ayurvedic application of spices delivers so much more than pleasant flavors. These potent and medicinal ingredients help us

- enhance and maintain good digestion,

- balance the doshas,

- incorporate all six tastes in a dish or a meal,

- transport nutrients from the food to the body's tissues,

- maintain an optimal metabolic rate,

- support the body's timely elimination functions, and

- maintain hormonal and emotional balance.

In *What to Eat for How You Feel*, I dedicated two chapters with detailed information on spices. In this chapter, I provide a quick reference to help you determine which spices would be most balancing for you today. Enjoy making my spice blend recipes (masalas), and use them as a guide to create your own.

SOURCING

Whenever purchasing spices from a grocery store or online, consider the following:

- Favor organic (not irradiated or fumigated) and recently harvested (check the packaging and expiration date).
- Buy whole spices because they have a longer shelf life (turmeric and asafoetida are exceptions).
- Purchase quantities proportional to your needs.

STORAGE AND USE

- Keep them in airtight, labeled containers (avoid plastic).
- Keep them in a dry, dark pantry or cupboard, away from light and moisture.
- Always use dry utensils for scooping.

DIGESTIBILITY

- Most spices require heat to activate their volatile compounds and make them bioavailable (peppercorns are an exception). It is best to cook with spices, and if you'd like to add them to uncooked items, such as salads, smoothies, or cold beverages, then dry toast the spices first.

COOKING TIPS

- Invest in a mortar and pestle and an electric spice grinder.
- Grind spices as needed for your meal, the week, or the month.
- When using an electric spice grinder, stop frequently to make sure that your spices don't overheat. The hotter the aroma molecules get, the more volatile they become—this lowers the intensity of flavor and medicinal properties.
- Combine heating spices with cooling ones to balance the overall effect on the body. For example, when using turmeric, ginger, or chiles, add fennel, coriander, or cilantro.

COOKING METHODS

- Dry toasting (e.g., Za'atar, page 234)
- Toast in fat (e.g., Turmeric Broth, page 238)
- Boiling (e.g., Quick Vegetable Broth, page 143)
- Paste (e.g., Creamy Spinach with Paneer Cheese, page 105)
- When toasting in fat, first heat the fat over low heat to a temperature conducive to frying (not smoking), then add spices in this sequence:
  1. largest pieces (e.g., cinnamon stick or bark, cardamom pods, dried bay leaves)
  2. ground turmeric—Vaidya Mishra taught me to add turmeric earlier than other ground spices because it needs a few extra seconds to activate; if the fat is very hot, add the ground turmeric last
  3. whole seeds (e.g., cumin, kalonji, ajwain, mustard, etc.)
  4. fresh spices (e.g., ginger, chile, curry leaves)
  5. ground spices (e.g., coriander, fennel, masalas)
  6. salt (exception is when cooking leafy greens or zucchini—for them, add salt toward the end of cooking because salt draws out water and can make your vegetables soggy)
- Cook with spices every day, and adjust the types and quantities for your dosha and seasonal balance needs.

COOLING SPICES	SLIGHTLY HEATING SPICES	HEATING SPICES
Use more in the summer but good all year round	Use all year round	Use more in the winter and spring
PITTA BALANCING AND TRIDOSHIC	TRIDOSHIC, BUT OMIT OR REDUCE IF PITTA IS HIGH	VATA AND KAPHA BALANCING
Caraway	Basil (some varieties)	Ajwain
Cardamom (green)	Bay Leaf	Allspice
Cilantro	Cinnamon	Asafoetida
Coriander	Cumin	Cardamom (black)
Dill	Curry Leaf	Chile
Fennel	Indian Bay Leaf	Clove
Mint	Nutmeg	Fenugreek
Rose	Parsley	Ginger (fresh and dry)
Sweet Basil	Rosemary	Kalonji
Tarragon	Saffron	Mace
Vanilla	Thyme (fresh)	Mustard (black, yellow/brown)
		Oregano
		Paprika
		Pepper (black, white, pink)
		Sumac
		Thyme (dried)
		Turmeric

warming masala

MAKES about ¼ cup ● PREP: 3 minutes ● GF, DF ● **FALL-WINTER-SPRING**

I learned this recipe from Vaidya R. K. Mishra. He combined one cooling and three heating spices to create a powerful blend that helps enhance digestion and clear the gut of *ama*. What's more—and some may argue more important—is the masala's great smell and taste.

Warming Masala goes well with any lentil dish, kitchari, leafy greens, and more.

1 tablespoon fennel seeds
1 tablespoon kalonji seeds
1 tablespoon ajwain seeds
1 tablespoon fenugreek seeds

1. Place all the ingredients in an electric spice grinder, and grind to a fine powder.

2. Store in an airtight jar away from light and humidity for up to 1 month.

protein digestive masala

MAKES about ¼ cup ● PREP: 5 minutes ● GF, DF ● **YEAR-ROUND**

Vaidya Mishra created this spice blend to support protein metabolism. I love using it with lentils, fresh cheese, kitchari, and sauces. It is a very balanced, tridoshic blend that you can cook with all year round.

2 tablespoons coriander seeds
2 tablespoons fennel seeds
2 teaspoons fenugreek seeds
1 teaspoon cumin seeds
1 teaspoon ground turmeric
1 teaspoon cardamom seeds
1 teaspoon cinnamon chips or
    ground cinnamon

1. Place all the ingredients in an electric spice grinder, and grind to a fine powder.

2. Store in an airtight container away from light and humidity for up to 1 month.

sweet masala #2

MAKES about 3 tablespoons • PREP: 5 minutes •
GF, DF • YEAR-ROUND

In *What to Eat for How You Feel*, I include a recipe for Sweet Masala, which is cooling to the physiology. This #2 blend is more warming but still balancing for all seasons. If your Pitta is very high, omit the black peppercorns.

1 tablespoon cinnamon chips or
   ground cinnamon
2 teaspoons coriander seeds
2 teaspoons fennel seeds
1 teaspoon vanilla powder
½ teaspoon cardamom seeds
8 black peppercorns
4 whole cloves

1. Place all the ingredients in an electric spice grinder, and grind to a fine powder.

2. Store in an airtight jar away from light and humidity for up to 1 month.

za'atar

MAKES about ½ cup • PREP: 10 minutes •
GF, DF • YEAR-ROUND

This beloved Middle Eastern blend comes in many versions, depending on the local culinary tradition. Regardless of the rendition, it is pungent and slightly tart, and it will help increase *agni*.

With this recipe, I show the dry-toasting method of cooking with spices. Since you toast some of the ingredients while making this recipe, this aromatic blend doesn't need much cooking when you apply it to a dish: add it toward the end of cooking or simply sprinkle it on cooked grains and vegetables (I love it with artichokes), salads, or toasted bread.

2 tablespoons white sesame seeds
¾ teaspoon cumin seeds
⅛ teaspoon salt
1 tablespoon dried thyme or savory
   (or half thyme and half marjoram)
1 tablespoon dried oregano
2 tablespoons sumac

1. Heat a small skillet over low heat, add the sesame seeds and cumin seeds, and toast until the sesame turns a light golden color. Immediately transfer to a grinding mortar, and let the seeds cool down.

2. Using the pestle, grind the toasted sesame seeds and cumin seeds with the salt until the seeds are mostly broken down. Add the thyme, and grind with a few more turns to mix it in, then add the oregano, and grind a bit more, until the spice blend is mixed well. Add the sumac, and stir with a spoon to mix well.

3. Store in an airtight container away from light and humidity for up to 1 month.

end-of-meal astringents

As I explain on page 25, ending your meal with something astringent sends a signal to your digestive system that the end of your meal is here.

Here are some ideas for end-of-meal astringent foods:

spiced buttermilk

Drink ½ cup buttermilk* blended with 1 tablespoon chopped fresh cilantro, ⅛ teaspoon toasted ground cumin, and a pinch of salt.

*This is the buttermilk derived from churning cultured cream into butter or from mixing whole plain yogurt with water (40:60 ratio).

honey

Lick a tiny spoonful of raw honey.

haritaki (*Terminalia chebula*)

Haritaki is a renowned fruit-herb in Ayurveda, used to open and clean clogged physical (and even mental) channels and to digest food. Although of predominant astringent taste, haritaki does not increase dryness in the body or aggravate Vata dosha. This herb is available at online Ayurvedic stores (see Sources, page 248).

Mix ⅛ teaspoon haritaki powder with one the following "carriers" for specific dosha balancing, and take it at the end of your meal:

DOSHA TO REDUCE	MIX WITH
Vata	¼ teaspoon melted cultured ghee
Pitta	¼ to ½ teaspoon powdered raw cane sugar
Kapha	a small pinch of Soma Salt
Tridoshic	½ teaspoon jaggery or honey

You may have a sip of warm water after taking the end-of-meal haritaki.

gentle detox tea

MAKES 4 cups ● PREP: about 12 minutes ●
GF, DF ● YEAR-ROUND

I learned this recipe from Vaidya Mishra. He advised using this tea when you experience high Pitta due to accumulated hot, acidic toxins in your liver or anywhere else in the body. He always stressed that such toxins should be cleansed away gently and slowly, and that is exactly what this tea does. The marshmallow root serves as a binder, to "package" the unwanted residue and promptly "ship" it out with the help of the remaining ingredients.

This tea is good for every body type. Make it first thing in the morning, sip a cup of it then, and store the rest in a thermos. Enjoy the remaining tea within four hours.

½ teaspoon fennel seeds
½ teaspoon coriander seeds
¼ teaspoon dried marshmallow root
2 fresh mint leaves or ¼ teaspoon dried mint

1. In a small saucepan, bring 4 cups filtered or spring water to a full boil, then turn off the heat. Add all of the ingredients, cover, and steep for 10 minutes. Strain the tea.

2. Store it in a thermos to keep it hot and sip slowly.

immune boost tea

MAKES 3 to 4 cups ● PREP: 5 minutes ●
COOK: 10 minutes ● GF, DF ● YEAR-ROUND

Here is a delicious Ayurvedic tea that acts both as a preventative and a relief for viral infections. It helps strengthen your body's defense system, and it reduces congestion and cough. It is also an excellent digestive aid for balancing any Vata and Kapha gut discomfort, like gas or bloating or heaviness. I made this tea a lot during the COVID-19 stay-at-home period in New York City. Even though my husband and I had no symptoms of infection, we would both relish this tea and think, "Ah, it's just what I needed."

3 tablespoons grated fresh ginger
4 green cardamom pods, slightly crushed open on one end
1 teaspoon fennel seeds
½ teaspoon ajwain seeds
Fresh lime or lemon juice to taste (about 1 tablespoon per cup)
Raw honey

1. In a small saucepan, combine 4 cups filtered or spring water, the ginger, cardamom pods, fennel seeds, and ajwain seeds, and bring to a boil over medium-high heat.

2. Partially cover, lower the heat to low, and simmer for 10 minutes.

3. Strain the tea. To serve, pour the tea into mugs, and let it cool down to sipping temperature, then stir in the lime juice and honey to taste. Sip slowly. If you'd like to keep it hot for a few hours, transfer it to a thermos.

Opposite (counterclockwise): Infused Olive Oil, Turmeric Broth, Gentle Detox Tea, Immune Boost Tea

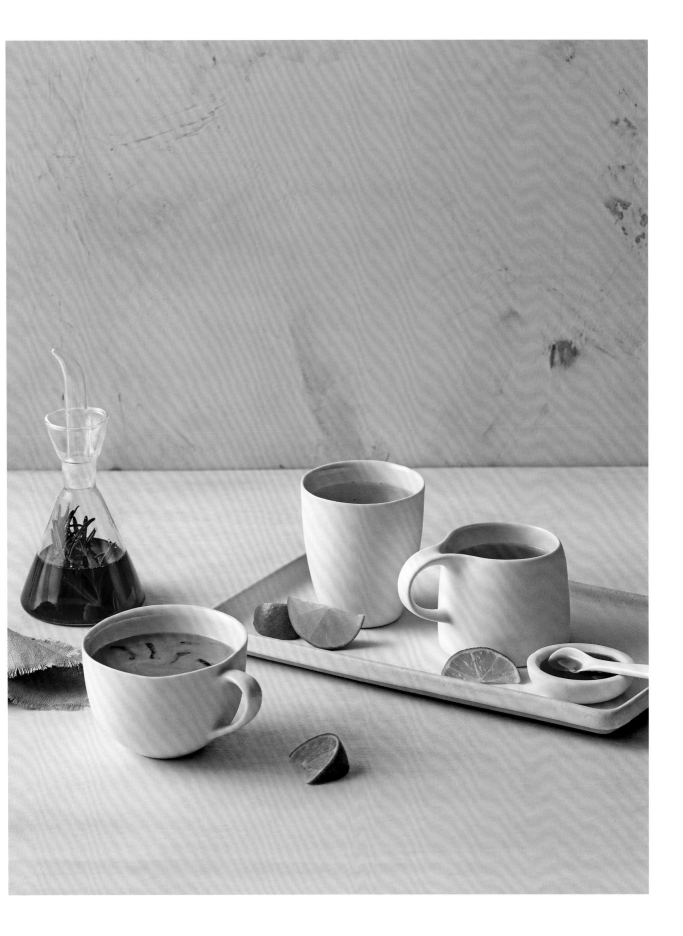

turmeric broth

MAKES about 1 cup ● PREP: 3 minutes ● COOK: about 5 minutes ● GF, DF ● YEAR-ROUND ●
Photograph on page 237

This recipe is perfect for when you're down with a cold or flu and feeling achy, congested, and without much of an appetite. It also works as a preventative for those conditions. More important, this broth does not taste like bitter medicine—it is delicious! All of the ingredients below have proven to have an anti-inflammatory and channel-opening effects on the body. Beet leaves in particular are rich in TMG (trimethylglycine), boasts numerous benefits, including support with liver detoxification and being a great source of antioxidants and energy.

My husband, Prentiss, deserves all the credit for creating this recipe based on the teachings of Vaidya R. K. Mishra.

1½ teaspoons ghee or olive oil

¼ teaspoon cumin seeds or black mustard seeds

½ teaspoon ground turmeric

¼ teaspoon fennel seeds

⅛ teaspoon ajwain seeds

2 teaspoons minced fresh ginger

1 small green Indian or Thai chile, seeded and minced (optional)

2 tablespoons whole fresh flat-leaf parsley leaves

2 tablespoons chopped beet leaves (optional)

¼ teaspoon salt, or to taste

1¼ cups boiling hot water

1 teaspoon fresh lime juice, or to taste

1. In a small saucepan, heat the ghee over medium-low heat, and add the cumin seeds. As soon as they turn gray and start to crackle, add the turmeric, fennel seeds, and ajwain seeds. Lower the heat to low, and toast the spices for about 5 seconds, until they release their aroma, then add the ginger and chile, and toast for a few more seconds; add the parsley, beet leaves, and salt. Sauté for about 10 more seconds, then pour in the hot water.

2. Cover and let the broth simmer over low heat for 3 minutes.

3. Serve the broth in a bowl, and let it cool down to sipping temperature, then add the lime juice. Sip slowly, and thoroughly chew the spices and the greens.

infused olive oil

MAKES about 1 cup ● **PREP:** 5 minutes ● **COOK AND COOL:** 35 minutes ● **GF, DF** ● **YEAR-ROUND** ●
Photograph on page 237

Here is yet another way for you to add a finishing touch of flavor to your salads, grains, vegetables, or cheese. Infused with a distinctive blend of herbs and spices, this oil lends a gentle aroma, color, and hint of pungency to lightly seasoned or unseasoned dishes. At Divya's Kitchen, we drizzle it over our Vegan Mozzarella Plate.

Use Infused Olive Oil for garnishing, not for cooking.

1 cup olive oil

1 teaspoon dried basil

1 teaspoon dried thyme or savory

1 teaspoon dried rosemary

1 teaspoon smoked paprika

¾ teaspoon salt

½ teaspoon dried oregano

2 green Indian or Thai chiles, seeded and minced

2 black cardamom pods, slightly crushed

⅛ teaspoon asafoetida

1. Pour the olive oil into a small dry saucepan. Start heating it over low heat, and add the remaining ingredients. When the oil starts to gently bubble, continue to simmer for another minute or two, until fragrant (do not allow it to reach a full boil!). Turn off the heat, and let the oil cool to room temperature, about 30 minutes.

2. Strain the oil through a fine-mesh strainer.

3. Store it in a clean, dry bottle with a tight-fitting cap. It will keep for up to two weeks in a dark cabinet or up to two months in the refrigerator.

nourish yourself

Dear reader,

Thank you for flipping through the pages of *Joy of Balance*. I hope my words and your making of the recipes give you clarity, confidence, and inspiration as you continue your healing with food. If you read about and experience firsthand the attributes of individual healing ingredients, I'm sure your relationship with food will evolve. The way you eat is deeply personal—not only can it be a source of enjoyment, but, more important, it is your source of sustenance, as your life depends on it; therefore, it is worth trying to change your eating habits for the better.

Improving anything in life, including our health, calls for shifting our perception to a place where balance aligns with life purpose. This may take years, but when you adjust your nourishment to support your life's journey, you will experience a sustained sense of joy and balance. You will feel integrated and content with life.

The Ayurvedic guidelines I share in this book are not absolute lines for *your* diet. Instead of obsessing over whether your meal is perfect, focus on turning your awareness to where you find balance. What does *your* health-promoting pattern of eating look like today?

Nourish yourself and let your fullness and happiness spill onto your family and friends. Meet frequently around the dining table, and express your love by cooking for them.

Let delicious food heal your body, mind, and relationships. Let everyone feel nourished.

With lots of love and gratitude,
Divya Alter

LET IT NOURISH YOU
—by my friend Dhyana Masla

We'll overeat
because we aren't allowing ourselves to
FULLY taste
what we're eating.

In the same way that you'll oversleep
if you aren't being rejuvenated from your sleep.

If we don't allow ourselves to be NOURISHED
by what we allow into our senses
then our senses are
constantly
craving
MORE.

(More sex,
more tv,
more food,
more sound, sight, taste, touch, smell.)

First, choose what truly NOURISHES YOU,
and then . . .
LET YOURSELF BE NOURISHED BY IT.

Meaning,
be present enough to not only touch but FEEL.
not only eat, but TASTE.
not only listen but HEAR.
not only smell but SAVOR.
not only look but SEE.

Invite your *attention*,
which invites what is *sacred*
into even the mundane.

Let yourself be nourished.

Let your practices
nourish you.

acknowledgments

This book came to life with the help of an expanded team of experts, friends, and family who generously contributed their time and talents to making my work substantially better.

At the onset, Leda Scheintaub, Renata Mihalic, Alyssa Benjamin, Franca Foligatti, and aunt Eleanor Hass helped me shape up the book proposal. Many thanks for getting me started on the right foot.

To my friends, Shyam-nam and Christian Halper: thank you for believing in me and my work and for your magnanimous support and encouragement.

I am most fortunate to have Ellen Scordato of Stonesong Publishing as my literary agent—thank you for your loving support and guidance.

To my Rizzoli publisher, Charles Miers, thank you for taking on my second book! Martynka Wawrzyniak, you shined again as my Rizzoli editor and supervised every single step of this book's manifestation. I'm also hugely grateful to you for bringing together the exceptional photography team: Rachel Vanni, a most skilled and tireless photographer; Caitlin Brown, the food stylist whose work excited me so much that I wanted to hug her for every image design; and Andrea Greco, the outrageously talented prop stylist who made me laugh or cry with joy on set—I will never forget that photo shoot with you all! Katie Eyles, you were instrumental in helping me shape up the manuscript and later proofread it. I owe you a vast debt of gratitude for spending countless hours on this and for being my writing mentor. Leda Scheintaub, I feel so lucky to have you as my copyeditor again. Your brilliance made the text infinitely better. Jan Derevjanik, I am in awe of your beautiful graphics and design work that make this book most attractive—thank you.

My heartfelt gratitude to all who assisted with the photo shoot: Katerina Martin, Renata Seear, Natasha Dayaramani, Melissa Neubert, Nandini Ravichandran, Kelly Spada, Kalpana Kanthan, Cynthia Kopyar, Jill Seymour, and Jess Palace. I could not have done all the sourcing and cooking without you.

I heartily thank our ANACT graduates who let me publish their recipes: Annie Mymokhod, Kandarpa Bhuckory, Bijal Shukla, Maria Torres, Federica Norreri, Andriy Egorovets, and Dhyana Masla for her beautiful poem.

The following friends and students assisted as text and recipe testers: Federica Norreri, Ryan Schmidt, Gina Tongonog, Valerie Hwang, Shubha Simhadri, Sasha Hynes, Ryann Morris, Katherine Banbury, Jahnavi Harisson, Palakh Chhabria, Dr. Bhaswati Bhattacharya, Cynthia Crumlish, Julia Alter, Carol Nace, Kandarpa Bhuckory, Gulnara Pugliese, Elliott Fredouelle, Susan Pack, Angelica Aroca, Marcia Baker, Mia Maria Westring, Kathleen Keating, and Meghan Alexandria (who also drafted the graphics in Part 1). Your candid feedback helped me refine the text and ensure that the recipes work—thank you all so much.

I feel most indebted to my Ayurveda teachers, Vaidya R. K. Mishra, Dr. Marianne Teitelbaum, Dr. Bhaswati Bhattacharya, Dr. John Douillard, Dr. Pratima Raichur, and Jai Dev Singh: your wisdom continues to transform my life and blossom my heart. The best way I can repay you is through service to you and others by sharing what I've learned from you.

I offer my deepest gratitude to my spiritual mentors, Krishna Kshetra Swami (Dr. Kenneth Valpey), Bhakti Tirtha Swami, and to my cooking mentor Yamuna Devi: thank you for your nurturing guidance and encouragement and for keeping me in line with my life's purpose.

My culinary students and Divya's Kitchen customers continue to inspire my deeper studies as well as recipe creations—this book is my expression of gratitude to you all.

My close family in Bulgaria cheered me on through every stage of the creation of this book— thank you, dear Mom, Dad, Sister, and Niece (Carla Fortuna). And in the US, thank you, Papa (Nick Alter) and Mom (Julia Alter) for your unconditional love. Finally, to the person I love deeply and with whom I get to celebrate life, my husband, Prentiss Alter: your affection, spirituality, charming demeanor, broad-minded intelligence, and generous heart make me laugh and grow every day. Thank you, thank you.

May this book bring joy and balance to all of you.

seasonal recipe guide

Here are suggestions for daily meals balanced both in nutrition and season. Many of my recipes can be made tridoshic—that is, balancing all year round. For guidance on this, read the dosha balancing variations under the recipe's ingredient list. * indicates to use in small amounts

Late Fall and Winter:
Warming and Vata
Balancing Meals

Adzuki Bean and Red
Lentil Patties (page 84)

Ayurvedic "Ketchup" (page 173)

Lime Rice Pilaf (page 65)

Steamed Kale Salad (page 109)

Immune Boost Tea (page 236)

———

Red Lentil and Celery Root Soup
(page 87)

Red Rice with Spinach and Nuts
(page 63)

Pistachio Fudge (page 187)

———

Celery Root and Taro Pancakes
(page 153)

Creamy Spinach with Paneer
Cheese (Palak Paneer) (page 105)

Plain Basmati Rice (page 64)

Green Tahini Sauce (page 219)

———

Asparagus Pizza (page 125)

Steamed Kale Salad (page 109)

Pineapple-Hibiscus Drink (page 168)

———

Cream of Fennel Soup (page 144)

Vegetable Bread (page 70)

Basil-Parsley Pesto (page 217)

———

Minestrone (page 51)

Vegan and Gluten-Free Bread
(page 57)

Basil-Parsley Pesto (page 217)

———

Dill-Mung Soup with Vegetable
Noodles (page 89)

Plain Basmati Rice (page 64)

Apple-Pear Turnovers with
Yacon "Caramel" Sauce (page 165)

———

Kulthi Lentil Stew, Puerto Rican
Style (page 81)

Ayurvedic "Ketchup" (page 173)

Plain Basmati Rice (page 64)

Gentle Detox Tea (page 236)

———

Cauliflower Soup with Almond
Cream (page 120)

Plain Basmati Rice (page 64)

Nori-Cheese Sticks (page 203)

Ayurvedic "Ketchup" (page 173)

———

Moroccan-Style Vegetable Tagine
(page 157)

Cashew Sour Cream (page 186)

Plain Basmati Rice (page 64)

Tamarind Sherbet (page 175)

———

Simple Kitchari (page 94)

Sweet Potato and Green Bean
Salad (page 151)

Green Tahini Sauce (page 219)

Immune Boost Tea (page 236)

———

Stuffed Cabbage Rolls (page 113)

Cashew Gravy (page 185)

Steamed Kale Salad (page 109)

Walnut-Orange Cake with
Honey Syrup (page 73)

Pineapple-Hibiscus Drink
(page 168)

———

Spring Greens Soup (page 108)

Marinated Paneer Cheese, Two
Ways (page 206)

Gluten-Free Paratha Flatbread
(page 56)

Green Tahini Sauce (page 219)

Immune Boost Tea (page 236)

———

Spring and Early Summer:
Cleansing and Kapha
Balancing Meals

Braised Purple Cabbage (page 117)

Millet Pilaf with Grated Carrots
(page 60)

Marinated Paneer Cheese,
Two Ways* (page 206)

———

Broccoli Rabe and Beets with
Saffron Almonds (page 102)

Gluten-Free Paratha Flatbread
(page 56)

Sautéed Mung Sprouts (page 92)

Immune Boost Tea (page 236)

———

Kulthi Lentil Stew, Puerto Rican
Style (page 81)

Plain Basmati Rice (page 64)

Ayurvedic "Ketchup" (page 173)

———

Minestrone (page 51)

Vegan and Gluten-Free Bread
(page 57)

Basil-Parsley Pesto (page 217)

———

Simple Kitchari (page 94)

Sautéed Bitter Melon (page 135)

Green Tahini Sauce (page 219)

Kulthi Tea (page 83)

———

Spring Greens Soup (page 108)

Sautéed Mung Sprouts (page 92)

Vegan and Gluten-Free Bread
(page 57)

———

ayurvedic food compatibility chart

Cheese

Ok to Combine with ...

Non-starchy vegetables: zucchini, asparagus, broccoli, radish, green beans

Leafy greens: Swiss chard, kale, collard greens, spinach

Nothing: may be eaten alone

Easy-to-digest lentils

Nuts

Bread, crackers, pasta (if digestion is strong)

Do NOT Combine in a Dish or a Meal with ...

Nightshades: eggplant, potatoes, peppers, tomatoes (if digestion is weak)

Eggs, milk, heavy cream

Meat, fish/seafood

Bread, crackers, pasta (if digestion is weak)

Heavy-to-digest beans: black, kidney, pinto, cannellini, lima

Fresh fruit

Yogurt

Ok to Combine with ...

Grains: wheat, rice, oats, amaranth, quinoa, millet, barley

Dried fruit: dates, raisins, figs, apricots, cranberries, currants, and more

Non-leafy vegetables: summer squash, cauliflower, broccoli, radish, cucumber

Nuts, seeds

Easy-to-digest lentils

All natural sweeteners, especially honey

Do NOT Combine in a Dish or a Meal with ...

Nightshades: eggplant, potatoes, peppers, tomatoes

Eggs

Milk, heavy cream

Leafy greens: Swiss chard, kale, collard greens, spinach

Fresh fruit, especially banana

Heavy-to-digest beans and lentils: black, kidney, pinto, cannellini, lima, urad dal

High heat: don't cook yogurt or buttermilk

Milk and Heavy Cream

Ok to Combine with ...

Grains: wheat, rice, oats, amaranth, quinoa, finger millet

Sweet dried fruit: dates, soaked raisins

Ghee, butter

Nuts, sunflower and pumpkin seeds

Spices: turmeric, ginger, black pepper, cinnamon, cardamom, cloves, saffron, vanilla, and more

Lentils: yellow split mung dal

Do NOT Combine in a Dish or a Meal with ...

Vegetables: leafy greens, radishes, nightshades (eggplant, potatoes, peppers, tomatoes), onions, garlic

Eggs, meat, fish/seafood, seaweed

Salt, sesame seed or paste

Fresh fruits: tree-ripened sweet mango and milk is an exception for a specific medicinal recipe

Sour/acidic foods: cheese, yogurt, buttermilk, citrus, alcohol, tomatoes, pickles, certain types of jaggery

Lentils and beans: kulthi, urad, chana, chickpeas, kitchari, and more

Grains: foxtail millet, barley

Yeasted breads, alcohol

Fresh Fruit

Ok to Combine with . . .

Nothing: best eaten alone,* at least 30 minutes before or 3 to 4 hours after a meal

*always true for melons

Fruits of the same kind and predominant taste: different kinds of berries, stone fruits and berries, apples and pears

Dates

Nuts and seeds: only true for citrus and other sour fruits

Nut and seed milk: almond, cashew, sunflower, oat

A lunch of proper food combinations: pineapple and papaya are the only exceptions to eating raw fruit with a meal due to their high enzymatic properties

Do NOT Combine in a Dish or a Meal with . . .

Dairy: milk, cream, yogurt, cheese, butter

Cooked foods

Raw vegetables

Grains

Lentils and beans

Leafy greens and salads

Do NOT Combine Radish with...

Jaggery, honey

Lotus stem

Bananas

Raisins

Milk

Urad dal

Do NOT Combine Cucumber with..

Lemon: use lime instead

Nightshades: potatoes, eggplant, tomatoes, peppers

Meat, Fish, or Eggs

Ok to Combine with . . .

Non-starchy vegetables: summer squash, cauliflower, broccoli, fennel, and more

Leafy greens: Swiss chard, kale, collard greens, spinach

Light side dishes: salad

Do NOT Combine in a Dish or a Meal with . . .

Dairy: milk, cream, yogurt, cheese, butter

Heavy foods: potatoes, pasta, bread, tortillas, beans and lentils (especially urad dal)

Honey

Sprouted pulses or grains

Each other: for example, meat and eggs

Alcohol (especially hard liquor)

Do NOT Combine Tapioca with...

Fruit: especially banana, mango, raisins

Heavy-to-digest beans: black, kidney, pinto, cannellini

Grains

Jaggery

Do NOT Combine Honey with...

Alcohol

Vegetables: water lily seed, radish

Chana dal/chickpeas

High heat: do not cook honey; allow foods and tea to cool slightly before adding

Rainwater

Ghee in equal proportions

glossary of terms and unfamiliar ingredients

AGNI: "That which engulfs"; the biological fire of digestion and metabolism governing all transformations in the organism; the solar energy component of *prana*.

AHARA: "That which we take in" with all our senses; food.

AHIMSA: Nonviolence; respect for all living things.

AJWAIN SEEDS: *Carum comticum*; a spice available in Indian and Middle Eastern grocery stores.

AMA: Undigested food; a cold and sticky unassimilated food matter that can cause blockages and inflammation.

AMA-VISHA: A type of toxicity in the body; reactive, hot, acidic *ama*.

ANJALI: An individual measurement for food portioning derived by holding one's two palms together like a bowl.

ARROWROOT (POWDER): *Maranta arundinacea*; a fine starch derived from the root of the arrowroot plant; a natural thickener and binder that is superior to cornstarch. Substitute two parts of arrowroot for one part cornstarch. Sold in health food stores.

ASAFOETIDA: *Ferula assa-foetida* (a.k.a. *hing*); a spice from the dried resin of an Indian plant; its strong sulfur aroma can replace the flavor of onions and garlic. Excellent, unadulterated quality is available at www.pureindianfoods.com. Use it in tiny quantities, as it can overheat the liver.

ASHRAM: A communal place for spiritual practice, such as yoga, prayer, and meditation.

ASHTANGA HRIDAYAM: One of the main Sanskrit classical texts on Ayurveda, by Vagbhata (assumed AD 550–600).

BESAN: The raw, untoasted flour of chana dal (easier to digest than garbanzo flour).

BHAVA PRAKASHA: One of the important Sanskrit classical works of Ayurveda, by Bhava Mishra (approximately AD sixteenth century).

CAMPHOR (EDIBLE): An extract from the camphor tree (*Cinnamomum camphora*); it has been used in many culinary traditions around the world. Available at Indian online grocery stores.

CHANA DAL: Hulled and split black chickpeas. Available in Indian grocery stores.

CHARAKA SAMHITA: One of the oldest, foundational Sanskrit texts of Ayurveda, presumed to be written by Charaka around 1000 BC.

CHENNA: Soft fresh cheese made by curdling milk and straining it without pressing. (See also page 201)

CURRY LEAVES: *Murraya koenigii* (a.k.a. sweet neem); a tropical and subtropical tree of which the leaves are used for cooking. Available in Indian grocery stores.

DGL POWDER: Ground deglycyrrhized licorice; an herb to cool down the liver and alleviate acidic digestion.

DOSHAS: Various combinations of the energies of ether, air, fire, water, and earth that perform all functions in the body; known as Vata, Pitta, and Kapha.

DRAVYA-GUNA-VIJNANA: The Ayurvedic pharmacology book compilation (in various editions and by many authors).

EINKORN: *Triticum monococcum*; the oldest and easiest to digest wheat known to humans. Sold at www.jovialfoods.com.

FENUGREEK SEEDS: *Trigonella foenum-graecum*; a spice useful for protein, fat, and sugar metabolism. Sold at health food stores and Indian grocery stores.

FIVE STATES OF MATTER (FIVE ELEMENTS): The elemental energies that are the building blocks of all material creation: ether, air, fire, water, and earth.

GARCINIA CAMBOGIA: Also known as *vrikshamla* in Sanskrit and *kodampuli* in Hindi. The fruit of the tree is used in cooking, spice and tea blends, and Ayurvedic remedies. It is of sour, pungent, and astringent tastes. It balances Vata and Kapha, increases *agni*, enhances the metabolic rate of the muscle and fat tissues, and optimizes circulation. Its cousin, *Garcinia Indica* (a.k.a. *kokum* in Hindi) has similar properties.

GREEN INDIAN OR THAI CHILE: *Capsicum annuum* (Thai chile a.k.a. bird's eye chile); small and very pungent chile sold in Asian grocery stores and health food stores. (See also page 220)

HARITAKI: *Terminalia chebula*; a medicinal fruit used in Ayurveda to correct many imbalances, such as toxic buildup, fatigue, premature aging, and more.

INDIAN BAY LEAF: *Cinnamomum tamala* (a.k.a. *tej patra* in Hindi); the leaf of the cinnamon tree used as a spice. Sold at https://divyas.com and in Indian grocery stores.

IRISH MOSS: *Gracilaria* (a.k.a. sea moss); type of red sea algae. Purchase the whole leaf at www.highvibe.com or www.essentialorganicingredients.com. (See also page 224)

JAGGERY: An Indian sweetener made by cooking down sugar cane juice until it thickens; it solidifies once it's cool.

KALONJI: *Nigella sativa* (a.k.a. black seed or black cumin); a spice sold at Indian grocery stores, https://divyas.com, and www.pure-indianfoods.com.

KAPHA: One of the three doshas that's represented by the energies of water and earth.

KASHA: Roasted buckwheat groats; sold in health food stores.

KULTHI LENTILS: *Macrotyloma uniflorum* (a.k.a. horse gram); a high-protein, low-calorie lentil used therapeutically in Ayurveda to break down calcification, stone, or tumor formations; clean the arteries; and more.

LEMON PEEL POWDER: A flavoring agent derived by drying and grinding lemon peels. Sold in Middle Eastern grocery stores and online.

MANJISHTHA: *Rubia cordifolia*; an Ayurvedic herb sold at www.chandika.com.

MARSHMALLOW ROOT (DRIED): *Althaea officinalis*; an herb used in cleansing protocols. Sold online or at health food stores.

MARUT: One of the three components of *prana*, composed of the cosmic space and air energies.

METABOLIC EFFECT (OF AN INGREDIENT): *Veerya;* an ingredient's power to bring about action or transformation in the body and thus produce a cooling, heating, or neutral effect on the liver.

OJAS: The essential by-product of all proper transformations in the body; the foundation for strong stamina and immunity.

PANEER CHEESE: Fresh cheese made by curdling milk, wrapping it in cheesecloth, and pressing it. (See also page 201.)

PITTA: One of the three doshas that's represented by the energies of fire and water.

POST-DIGESTIVE EFFECT: *Vipaka*; the end-transformation of the six tastes of food as it becomes absorbed in the body. There are three post-digestive effects: sweet, sour, and pungent.

PRAKRITI: A person's inherent nature or body-mind constitution, expressed as unique proportions of the Vata, Pitta, and Kapha doshas.

PRANA: The life-giving energy that circulates in the environment and in every living being; the cosmic energy that carries the potential of matter.

PSYLLIUM HUSK POWDER: *Plantago ovata*; the ground version of the seed's husks; it is known as a prebiotic and digestive; acts as a binder in gluten-free baking. Sold in the supplements section in health food stores.

PURANAS: A genre of ancient Indian encyclopedic literature covering diverse topics in all areas of life.

QUINOA FLAKES: Pressed quinoa seeds; sold in health food stores.

ROSE WATER: The by-product of distilling rose petals into oil; look for the edible or food grade kind in health food stores, usually in the skin care department.

SATTU: The flour of dry-roasted chana dal. Available in Indian grocery stores.

SHAKA VANSIYA LINEAGE: Also know as Shaka-vamsha or the lineage of the people from the land of the Śakas, mentioned in the *Samba Purana* (AD 650–850); an old, continuous, and living tradition of Ayurvedic knowledge. Vaidya R. K. Mishra brought this tradition to the US and then made it known throughout the world by innovating and adapting Ayurveda to the new circumstances and new types of patients, while at the same time maintaining the integrity of the Shaka Vansiya's distinctive approach both in theory and in practice.

SOMA: One of the three components of *prana*, composed of the cosmic lunar energy.

SOMA SALT: A brand name for *saindhava*; a type of whitish rock salt sourced from the Sindh region in Pakistan. Ayurveda considers it the best type of salt because it has a cooling metabolic effect and decreases high blood pressure; sold at https://divyas.com and www.chandika.com

SUMAC: *Rhus coriaria*; a tangy, red spice derived by grinding the dried fruits of the sumac shrub. Sold in Middle Eastern grocery stores and online.

SUNFLOWER LECITHIN: Extracted by cold-pressing the gum of the sunflower plant; an excellent substitute for soy lecithin, which is commonly produced from genetically modified soybeans. It generates emulsifying and lubricating effects in food preparations; sold in health food stores.

SUSHRUTA SAMHITA: One of the oldest Sanskrit texts of Ayurveda, by Sushruta (approximately 600 BC).

SWEET TAMARIND: *Tamarindus indica*; the sweet variety of the tamarind tree. Fresh pods are sold in both common grocery stores and health food stores as Sweet Thai Tamarind. (See also page 171.)

TARO ROOT: *Colocasia esculenta*; a tropical tuber common in warm-climate cuisines throughout the world; sold in Indian and Asian grocery stores. (See also page 152.)

TRIDOSHIC: Balancing for all three doshas; a person whose constitution is made of equal proportions of the three doshas.

VATA: One of the three doshas that's represented by the energies of ether and air.

VEDAS: A large body of the oldest Sanskrit texts originating in India; they were transmitted orally long before they were written around 1500 BC. Corollary to the *Vedas*, there is a vast corpus of Vedic texts, such as the *Samhitas* and *Upanishads*.

YACON SYRUP: A sweetener extracted from the tuberous yacon plant. It is very nutritious and low glycemic, and it helps decrease body weight.

sources

Divya's

https://divyas.com
Divya's Kitchen (restaurant), classes, videos, certification program, recipes, and more
Online Store: Our line of ready-to-go meal packets, cultured ghee, Soma Salt, spices, Divya's cookbooks, and more

Ingredients and Products

Chandika
https://chandika.com
High-quality Ayurvedic remedies, personal care products, and culinary ingredients formulated by Vaidya R.K. Mishra

Pure Indian Foods
https://pureindianfoods.com
Organic yellow split mung dal, chana dal, besan, cultured ghee, rose water, spices, and more

High Vibe
https://highvibe.com
Organic Irish moss, high-quality olive oil, coconut oil, seaweed, and more

Fandango Olive Oil
https://fandangooliveoil.com
Divya's favorite US brand of high-quality olive oil

Amphora Nueva
https://amphoranueva.com
The freshest high-quality olive oil from around the world

Jedwards International
https://bulknaturaloils.com/
Yacon syrup, oils, and more

Jovial Foods
https://jovialfoods.com
Organic einkorn (berries, flour, pasta), gluten-free flour blends

Pratima Skin Care and Spa
https://pratimaskincare.com
Ayurvedic skin care and spa treatments

Life Spa
https://lifespa.com
Herbal supplements, articles, podcasts, and consultations by Dr. John Douillard, DC

Gita Nagari Eco Farm and Sanctuary
http://theyogafarm.com
Cruelty-free dairy products and adopt-a-cow and organic CSA programs

Equipment

Ancient Cookware
https://ancientcookware.com
Traditional Ayurvedic clay pots and nontoxic natural cookware (such as tagine pots)

Pleasant Hill Grain
https://pleasanthillgrain.com
KoMo grain mills and flakers, spice grinders, and other kitchen appliances

Ayurveda Knowledge and Training

Divya's
https://divyas.com
Divya's classes, videos, certification program, recipes, and more

SV Ayurveda
https://svayurveda.com
Archived articles by Vaidya R.K. Mishra, recorded and live courses, recipes, and more

The DINacharya Institute
http://dinacharya.org
Masterclasses and training with Dr. Bhaswati Bhattacharya and other Ayurveda teachers

Dr. Marianne Teitelbaum
https://drmteitelbaum.com/online-classes/
Ten free 1+ hour-long classes and other videos on various health topics from the perspective of SV Ayurveda

Life-Force Academy
https://teachings.jaidevsingh.com
Classes and courses on yoga, dharmic business, Ayurveda for beginners, and more, led by Jai Dev Singh

Ayurvedic Consultations/ Integrative Medicine

Dr. Marianne Teitelbaum, DC
https://drmteitelbaum.com

Dr. Bhaswati Bhattacharya, MD
http://drbhaswati.com

Dr. Robert E. Graham, MD
https://freshmednyc.com

Dr. Gulnara Pugliese, MD
http://drpugliesemd.com

Body Type/Dosha Quizzes

By Jai Dev Singh
https://activate.jaidevsingh.com/ayurveda-quiz-course-owners/

By Dr. John Douillard, DC
https://lifespa.com/ayurvedic-health-quizzes/dosha-body-type-quiz-form/

digestion questionnaire

In each section, mark or check the questions to which your answer is "yes." Tally up your responses. The section with the most "yes" answers is likely an accurate indication of your current state of digestion.

Imbalanced—
Irregular/Vata/Airy

○ Is your appetite up and down?

○ Do you have frequent bloating, distention, or gas?

○ Do you experience churning and gurgling in your stomach?

○ Do you have low energy, especially in the afternoons?

○ Do you have frequent hiccups or belching without acid after meals?

○ Do you experience hoarseness or dryness in your mouth or in your speech?

○ Do you often have the urge to pass stool but cannot?

○ Do you have constipation or irregular, hard, dry stools?

○ Do you retain urine or urinate too much?

○ Do you have problems maintaining or gaining weight?

○ Do you have cracking and loose joints?

○ Do you have dry, scaly skin?

○ Are your hands and feet frequently cold?

Imbalanced—
Sharp/Pitta/Fiery

○ Do you have uncontrollable hunger and need to eat immediately?

○ Do you have frequent hyperacidity and heartburn?

○ Do you have bad smelling breath?

○ Do you have a tendency toward nausea?

○ Do you have a craving for sweets or cold food?

○ Do you frequently wake up around two in the morning feeling hungry?

○ Do you experience night sweats or excessive sweating and body heat?

○ Do you experience frequent grief and sadness without a reason?

○ Do you feel emotionally oversensitive?

○ Do you tend to feel a burning sensation in your eyes and eyelids?

○ Are your eyes red and easily irritated?

○ Are your eyes sensitive to light?

○ Do you experience burning and itching on your skin and scalp?

○ Are you prone to hives and rashes?

○ Do you have frequent pimples, pustules, or skin infections?

○ Do you get scaly, red lesions on your skin (e.g., eczema, psoriasis)?

Imbalanced—
Slow/Kapha/Earthy

○ Do you lack appetite, often feeling full and heavy in the stomach?

○ Do you feel sluggish after eating?

○ Do you have excessive or insufficient saliva?

○ Do you have a lack of or distorted taste?

○ Is your tongue coated with a white film in the morning?

○ Do you have excessive phlegm?

○ Do you have a feeling of heaviness in the head?

○ Are you overweight, or do you gain weight easily?

○ Do you have nausea with vomiting of mucus?

○ Do you frequently get colds, coughs, or congestion?

○ Do you have swelling or stiffness of the joints?

○ Do you have oily skin, a tendency toward sebaceous cysts, lipoma (fatty tumor), or skin buildup?

Balanced—
The Ideal

○ Do you get hungry at regular times, about four hours after each meal?

○ Do you feel satiated yet light and energized after eating?

○ Do you maintain good energy throughout the day without caffeine?

○ Is your tongue clear of a white coating in the morning?

○ Do you have a regular, well-shaped bowel movement first thing in the morning and possibly again in the evening?

○ Do you effortlessly maintain your optimal weight?

○ Do you have clear, glowing skin?

○ Do you often get compliments that you look much younger than your age?

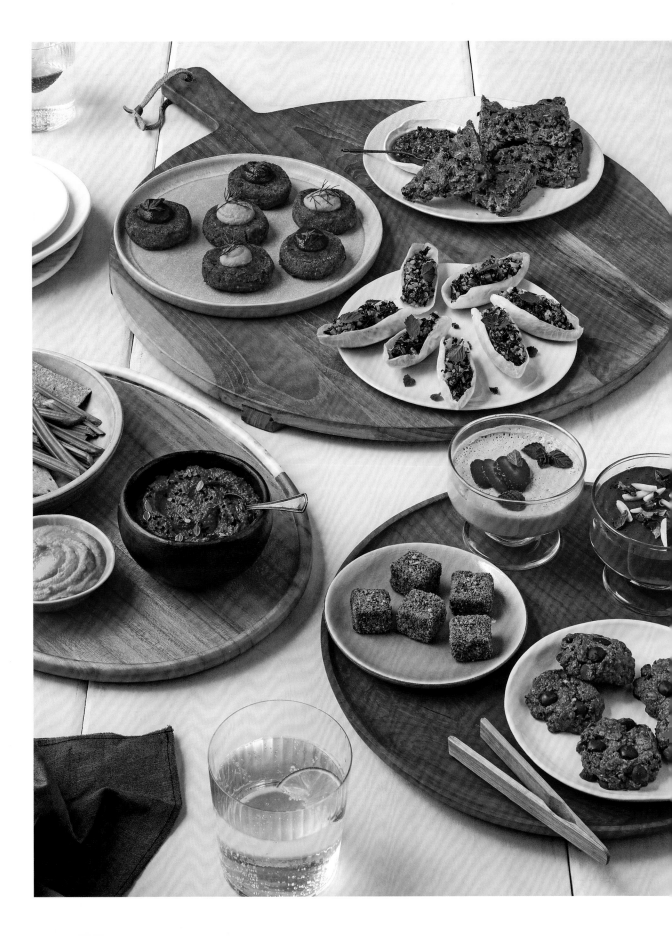

index

Opposite: Finger Foods for the Party Table (clockwise): Adzuki Bean and Red Lentil Patties with Roasted Carrot Tahini Sauce and Ayurvedic "Ketchup," Vegetable Bread with Basil-Parsley Pesto, Green Tabbouleh in yellow endive boats; Strawberry Parfait, Rose Chocolate Mousse, Pecan Chocolate Chip Cookies, Pistachio Fudge, Sunflower-Beet Hummus, Roasted Carrot Tahini Sauce, Sesame Crackers with celery sticks

First published in the United States of America in 2022
by Rizzoli International Publications, Inc.
300 Park Avenue South
New York, NY 10010
www.rizzoliusa.com

Publisher: Charles Miers
Author: Divya Alter
Editor: Martynka Wawrzyniak
Production Manager: Kaija Markoe
Managing Editor: Lynn Scrabis
Designer: Jan Derevjanik

Photographer: Rachel Vanni
Food Stylist: Caitlin Haught-Brown
Prop Stylist: Andrea Greco

2022 2023 2024 2025/ 10 9 8 7 6 5 4 3 2 1

Distributed in the U.S. trade by
Random House, New York

Printed in China

ISBN: 9780847872404

Library of Congress Control Number: 2022935017

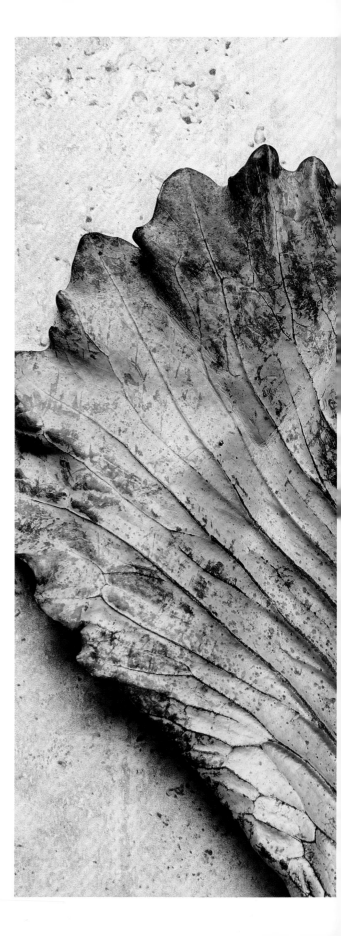